Visit our website

to find out about more books from Churchill Livingstone
and other Harcourt Health Sciences imprints

Register free at
www.harcourt-international.com

and you will get

- the latest information on new books, journals and electronic products in your chosen subject areas

- the choice of e-mail or post alerts or both, when there are any new books in your chosen areas

- news of special offers and promotions

- information about products from all Harcourt Health Sciences imprints including W. B. Saunders, Churchill Livingstone, and Mosby

You will also find an easily searchable catalogue, online ordering, information on an extensive list of journals...and much more!

Visit the Harcourt Health Sciences website today!

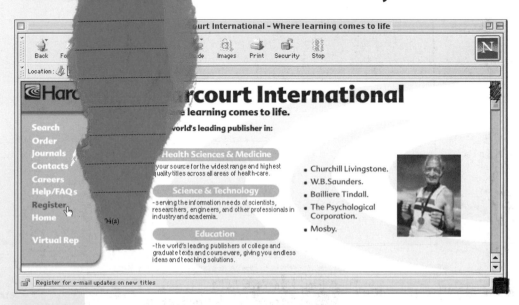

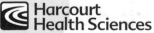

Occupational Therapy for Child and Adolescent Mental Health

For Churchill Livingstone:

Editorial Director: Mary Law
Project Development Manager: Katrina Mather
Project Manager: Jane Shanks
Design Direction: George Ajayi

Occupational Therapy for Child and Adolescent Mental Health

Edited by

Lesley Lougher BSc SOC Dip COT
Community CAMHS Manager, North West Anglia Healthcare Trust, Peterborough, UK

Foreword by

Linda L. Florey PhD OTR FAOTA
Chief, Rehabilitation Services, UCLA Neuropsychiatric Institute, Los Angeles, USA

Cartoons by
Deborah Hutton Dip COT
Head Occupational Therapist, Family Consultation Service,
North West Anglia Healthcare Trust, Peterborough, UK

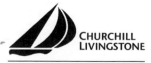

CHURCHILL
LIVINGSTONE

EDINBURGH LONDON NEW YORK PHILADELPHIA ST LOUIS SYDNEY TORONTO 2001

CHURCHILL LIVINGSTONE
An imprint of Harcourt Publishers Limited

© Harcourt Publishers Limited 2001

 is a registered trademark of Harcourt Publishers Limited

The right of Lesley Lougher to be identified as editor of this work has been asserted by her in accordance with the Copyright, Designs and Patents Act 1988

First published 2001

ISBN 0 443 06134 3

British Library Cataloguing in Publication Data
A catalogue record for this book is available from the British Library

Library of Congress Cataloging in Publication Data
A catalog record for this book is available from the Library of Congress

Note
Medical knowledge is constantly changing. As new information becomes available, changes in treatment, procedures, equipment and the use of drugs become necessary. The editor, contributors and the publishers have taken care to ensure that the information given in this text is accurate and up to date. However, readers are strongly advised to confirm that the information, especially with regard to drug usage, complies with the latest legislation and standards of practice.

The
publisher's
policy is to use
paper manufactured
from sustainable forests

Printed in China

Contents

Chapter Opening Cartoons: Deborah Hutton tracks the progress of a family through subjects of the chapters.

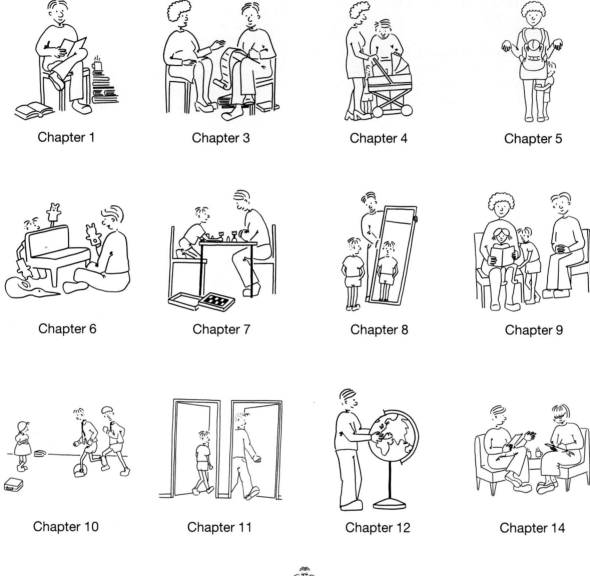

Chapter 1

Chapter 3

Chapter 4

Chapter 5

Chapter 6

Chapter 7

Chapter 8

Chapter 9

Chapter 10

Chapter 11

Chapter 12

Chapter 14

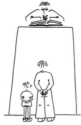

Chapter 15

Contributors

Pauline Blunden Dip COT SROT

Senior Occupational Therapist, Child and Adolescent Mental Health Service, The Child Health Centre, Bury St Edmonds, Suffolk, UK

Ann Christie Dip OT NZROT FRLA 1998

Senior Occupational Therapist/Clinical Specialist, Child Mental Health, Community Child Adolescent and Family Service and Triple A Team, Starship Hospital, 76 Grafton Road, Private Bag 92024, Grafton, Auckland, New Zealand. Email: Achristie@ahsl.co.nz and tanekaha@powerlink.co.nz

Becky Durant BEd(Hons) Post Grad Dip Mental Health Dip COT

Head Occupational Therapist/Clinical Specialist, Bethel Child and Family Centre, Mary Chapman House, Norwich, UK

Alan Evans BA(Hons) Dip COT Post Grad Dip Art therapy

Head Occupational Therapist, Oakham House, Adolescent Unit, Leicester, UK

Sue Evans Dip COT SROT

Senior Occupational Therapist, Leigh House Adolescent Psychiatric Hospital, Winchester, UK

Anna Flanigan Dip COT

Former Senior Occupational Therapist, Iddesleigh House Clinic, Exeter; now child Therapist, Joint Agency Child Abuse Team (JACAT), Exeter; Student Counsellor, Exeter College, Course Tutor, Diploma in Counselling, University of Exeter, UK

Carol Hardy Dip COT MA

Head Occupational Therapist/Clinical Specialist, Under Eights Service, Bloomfield Centre, Guy's Hospital, London, UK

Gita Ingram Dip COT SROT

Head Occupational Therapist, Child and Family Mental Health Service, Lothian Primary Care NHS Trust, Edinburgh, UK

Laurette J. Olson MA

Doctorial Candidate, New York University, Instructor in Occupational Therapy, Mercy College, Occupational Therapy Consultant, Mamaroneck Union Free School District, New York, USA

Sue Pownall

Head Occupational Therapist, Child and Family Guidance, Central Health Clinic, Southampton, UK

Karin Prior BSc OT MA

Senior Occupational Therapist, Under Eights Service, Bloomfield Centre, Guy's Hospital, London, UK

Rowena Scaletti NZROT MHSc (Occupational Therapy) CertArts (Sociology) Postgrad Dip Ed (Counselling)

Family Therapist, Bapist Action Services, PO Box 98840 FANC Wiri, South Auckland, New Zealand

Foreword

Occupational Therapy for Child and Adolescent Mental Health is the first occupational therapy book in both the UK and the USA to provide a comprehensive view of occupational therapy mental health practice for children and adolescents. Typically, occupational therapy textbooks devote a chapter or a few pages to this area of practice or they focus on only one disorder such as autism. Occupational therapy for children and adolescents with behavioural and emotional difficulties has not achieved prominence in practice or in publications in either the UK or the USA. In 1989, I became convinced that these children were not addressed by occupational therapists working with either children or mental health populations and furthermore, that psychosocial aspects of child behaviour were being ignored (Florey 1989). The issue is not that children do not experience problems in social and emotional domains. They are hidden in plain sight and their needs are becoming more apparent as instances of youth violence achieve international prominence. This textbook is timely and it provides an excellent first step in addressing this important practice area.

Lougher authors the first two chapters which ground the reader in the issues of services for children and adolescents and provide a scholarly review of practice in this area. More importantly, Lougher raises key issues for examination and provides challenges to therapists practising in this area. One challenge is framed politically, the other clinically: she reasons that if occupational therapists view people as social beings and as initiators of action, they must also pay attention to the social context of their own practice. It is not sufficient for occupational therapists to say they make a difference in treatment or to continue to dwell only in direct service provision. They must stand up and advocate for inclusion in the service delivery system. She rightfully argues that occupational therapy has an obligation to become involved in the political climate in which service systems are generated and to advocate for occupational therapy services to benefit children. The political challenge is to identify core occupational therapy services and to advocate for these services by affecting the larger health care system at the policy level.

The second challenge is that occupational therapists must stand by the core of their practice and shed the cloak of invisibility. Lougher suggests that part of the invisibility is self imposed in that occupational therapists have so blended their focus in the guise of teamwork that their service is indistinguishable from that of another team member. The team is invaluable but the core expertise of each member must be celebrated, not blended. Blended evaluations and blended treatment dilute the unique skills of each team member and the result is often mediocre practice by all. Another level of invisibility occurs as therapists take on specialist skills and then prefer to practice these skills or identify themselves by the specialty while neglecting the core skills of occupational therapy. The clinical challenge is to identify the core knowledge and fundamental skills upon which occupational therapy rests and to demonstrate this through assessment and treatment.

The challenges Lougher raises are by no means unique to this area of practice nor to the UK. They represent the changing strategies for patient care that therapists must adopt which demand a clear understanding of the core principles of occupation on which occupational therapy rests. It will always be necessary for occupational therapists to struggle with the complexity inherent in the seemingly simple idea of occupation. This is the challenge occupational science has undertaken.

The book is divided into five sections, each of which targets a different focus for consideration. Section 1 acquaints the reader with services for children and adolescents with behaviour and emotional difficulties and provides an overview of the major diagnostic categories seen in child mental health. Lougher describes the background and changes in service delivery within Child and Adolescent Mental Health Services (CAMHS) and locates these services within the broad historical context of service in the UK. She acquaints the reader with the key components of the four-tiered approach to delivery of CAMHS in the UK and the existing or potential contributions of occupational therapy at each tier. She strongly advocates the need for occupational therapists to claim and practice within the core skills of occupational therapy and suggests a template for this core based upon occupation. Evans (Ch. 3) reviews prevalence and key symptoms of the most frequently encountered psychiatric disorders seen within the child and adolescent population.

Section 2 acquaints the reader with the various frames of reference that inform practice. The intent of this section is to provide sufficient review of theoretical approaches such that a practitioner new to the field is informed of the key interdisciplinary perspectives in this area. Pownall (Ch. 4) reviews major developmental perspectives which serve as a foundation for understanding abnormal behaviour. Hardy and Prior (Ch. 5) review the origins and classification of attachment behaviour and attachment issues at different ages while Blunden (Ch. 6) depicts the varied perspectives on the therapeutic use of

play. Durant (Ch. 7) discusses family therapy, systems theory, and the model of human occupation and Ingram (Ch. 8) concludes this section with a review of classic psychodynamic theories.

Section 3 describes current occupational therapy practice in the UK according to and with emphasis on developmental level. Hardy (Ch. 9) summarizes the key issues to be considered in working with infants and children up to five years of age and focuses on the interpersonal context in which problems with young children arise. Prior (Ch. 10) highlights work with school-aged children and discusses the changing nature of competencies and relationships with peers and adults as children enter school life. She stresses the therapeutic value of play and work, and motivational and safety issues with this age group and discusses focal points in structuring therapeutic activities. Flanigan (Ch. 11) provides a brief overview of developmental issues in adolescence and reviews different methods of assessment, the range of therapeutic interventions, and focuses on group work with this population.

Section 4 highlights the focus of occupational therapy mental health services with children and adolescents from an international perspective which includes the USA and New Zealand. Olson (Ch. 12) offers a cogent view of the issues in occupational therapy practice in the USA. She reviews implications of the health service delivery system and the move within the profession to renew allegiance to the core value of occupation in practice. Christie and Scaletti (Ch. 13) discuss the multicultural heritage of New Zealand, and the changing health care system and consequent need for occupational therapy to redefine practice. They list prominent treatment approaches, models and theories, and frames of reference used in New Zealand and provide examples of occupational therapy practice focus.

Section 5 includes two areas that underlie practice: supervision and knowledge of laws affecting children. Evans (Ch. 14) discusses the need for supervision and support for occupational therapists working with this population of children and adolescents, particularly as therapists often practice in departments in which they are isolated from other occupational therapists. Durant

(Ch. 15) reviews the main principles of protective legislation for children including the Children Act, the Mental Health Act, and the Education Act and implications of these acts for occupational therapists.

This book should be widely read as it is valuable to practitioners in the field and to those wishing to enter this area of practice. The fundamental knowledge of development with a psychosocial focus also provides a foundation for practitioners who work with children with a variety of medical and neurological disorders as well.

I applaud the contributors to this important first book in child and adolescent mental health and I look forward to occupational therapists in the UK and the USA rising to the political and clinical challenges set forth by Lougher.

Los Angeles 2000   Linda L. Florey

REFERENCE

Florey L 1989 Treating the whole child: rhetoric or reality? American Journal of Occupational Therapy 43(6): 365–369

Preface

Occupational therapists work in all areas of child and adolescent mental health services (CAMHS) but from reading the literature they are almost invisible. This book aims to demonstrate the contribution made by occupational therapists to clinical practice in CAMHS teams. Each chapter is written by a practising occupational therapist with many years' experience in CAMHS. I hope to suggest that occupational therapists have opportunities to develop programmes at all levels of the service, from early intervention, working with primary care teams, to residential units.

The book arises from a course I organised for the National Association of Paediatric Occupational Therapists (NAPOT) in 1996, to introduce occupational therapists to this field of work. Most of the authors here contributed to that event. As an occupational therapist with, then, 14 years' experience in CAMHS, the depth of experience and knowledge within the profession impressed me. The authors would not claim that only occupational therapists use the theories and therapies described here, but we do believe that our profession has a particular way of interpreting and using them.

The contributions from the USA and New Zealand add an extra dimension to this exploration of occupational therapy in CAMHS, in the description of the service context as well as in forms of therapeutic intervention. The occupational therapy theory of sensory processing and integration gets but a passing mention by the British authors, although it may be used more widely as greater links are developed between paediatric services and CAMHS.

All the contributors are experts in their fields with many years of experience and further study. Each chapter is written in the style that follows from the theory described, as occupational therapists attracted to this area of work need to learn the language their colleagues will use.

This overview of the range of approaches used in one area of work provides a snapshot of the ingenuity of the profession and should be of interest to both undergraduate and practising occupational therapists in CAMHS, paediatrics and adult mental health services.

Northamptonshire 2000   Lesley Lougher

Preface

Acknowledgements

I would like to thank the following for making this book possible:

My father, who suggested the career of occupational therapy but died before this book was published.

My long-suffering husband, who cooked, gardened and gave IT support, whilst I grappled with this enormous project I had taken on so lightly.

Deborah Hutton, who not only drew the illustrations, but was the first occupational therapist to join me in Peterborough and has contributed to the development of my ideas.

NAPOT for enabling me to meet so many occupational therapists working in CAMHS.

Introduction

1

SECTION CONTENTS

Over the past few years, Child and Adolescent Mental Health Services (CAMHS) have received more attention from government, agencies working with children and media than at any time in their history. Section 1 aims to introduce the reader to services for children who are experiencing behavioural and emotional difficulties. Chapter 1 describes some of the recent changes so that readers are able to understand the context of occupational therapy practice in this field. The content of this practice over 30 years is examined in Chapter 2, by considering the literature published in the occupational therapy press in Britain and the USA. An overview of the types of problems and disorders encountered in CAMHS is outlined by Alan Evans in Chapter 3.

1

Introduction to child and adolescent mental health services

Lesley Lougher

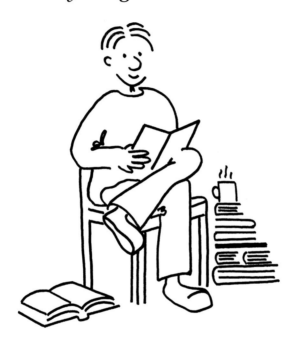

INTRODUCTION

Occupational therapy is rarely mentioned in the child psychiatry literature. Some responsibility for this omission rests with the profession. Many occupational therapists have worked as single-tons in multidisciplinary teams and have merged their professional identity in a generic team. Publication and research has not been high on the agenda in this practice-based profession as a whole. There have been some notable exceptions in the UK, such as Lily Jeffrey who wrote about occupational therapy in child and adolescent mental health services (CAMHS) in the 1980s, followed by others from Newcastle, more recently

Telford and Ainscough. Individually occupational therapists are seen as valuable team members, but not as belonging to a specific profession.

Occupational therapy is a relatively small profession numerically, compared with nursing, and has few statutory powers compared with medicine and social work, and less ability in self-promotion than psychology. Mental health services have in the past been the poor relation compared with acute physical services, and CAMHS was the Cinderella of the mental health services. In the UK, occupational therapy became the Cinderella profession in the Cinderella service.

Times have changed for CAMHS. The Health Advisory Service report (1995) *Together We Stand* drew attention to the crisis in CAMHS and governmental concerns about children's ability to achieve and fears about youth crime put the welfare of young people on to the political agenda. In a climate where a price was placed on healthcare services, professions and services have needed to prove their effectiveness. Greater awareness has arisen as to the areas of difference between professions rather than the degree of overlap, so that occupational therapists have begun to contact one another to compare practice and gain support.

In the 1980s Jeffrey's survey located 82 occupational therapists in post in child psychiatric units. (Jeffrey, Lyne & Redfern 1984). By 1998 10% of the 1000 members of the National Association of Paediatric Occupational Therapists stated that they were working in CAMHS and there are many others who are not members.

One of the philosophical assumptions of occupational therapy is a view of people as social beings and initiators of action (Creek 1997) so that the social context is central to the therapeutic process. Occupational therapists do not always apply this understanding to the context of their own work and so are unaware of changes in national and local policies. If there is a belief that occupational therapy brings a unique understanding to the promotion of mental health, then therapists have an obligation to ensure their views are represented. It is not sufficient to focus only on the delivery of effective therapy and to

hope that virtue will be rewarded by recognition from policy-makers. Just as clients are encouraged to take an active role in the design of the treatment plan, so occupational therapists need to be aware of the process of decision-making both locally and nationally. Development of services is dependent on the ability to attract additional funding which is released in order to meet governmental targets.

This is an important time for child and adolescent mental health services (CAMHS) as there is governmental recognition of the need to ensure that the nation's children receive a better start in life if they are to become healthy adults. There are also significant opportunities for occupational therapists to promote the value of their contribution to this area of work. A better understanding of the present is gained when placed in context of the past.

A BRIEF HISTORY OF CAMHS

Recognition of the mental health needs of children has emerged during the twentieth century, although there are records of adolescents being admitted into the private 'madhouses' and asylums in the eighteenth and nineteenth centuries. In Britain, the School Medical Service was established in 1907, with a remit of medico-sociological work concerned with a wide range of disorders (Parry Jones 1989). Anna Freud and Melanie Klein began treating children with psychoanalysis in the 1920s. Freud moved to London in 1938 to become the director of two wartime day nurseries (Sayers 1991).

In Britain child psychiatry emerged as a sub-specialty of adult psychiatry in the 1930s. Child psychiatrists were influenced strongly by the mental hygiene movement, the aim of which was to prevent disturbance in adults (Graham 1994). Child Guidance Clinics were established around the same time, to provide a community-based interdisciplinary service, staffed by psychiatrists, psychiatric social workers and educational psychologists. The theoretical approach of child guidance was concerned with 'adjusting the growing individual to his own immediate environment' rather than the curing of mental illness

(Parry Jones 1989). The clinic staff frequently used a psychoanalytical frame of reference, where either the psychiatrist or the psychologist treated the child and a psychiatric social worker worked with the mother, fathers perhaps being seen as peripheral to the process.

Residential units for children and adolescents were often attached to large mental hospitals and many were organised along the principle of a therapeutic community. Provision for adolescents with acute mental health problems have always been less common. Occupational therapists are mentioned in the literature in the 1950s (Rockey 1987) working in 'psychological' hospitals for children. Forward wrote about her treatment of disturbed and psychotic children in 1953 and 1958 (Rockey 1987).

The concept of the multiagency Child Guidance Clinic faded. First of all the educational psychologists were withdrawn, so that by 1990 there were none reported working in child and adolescent mental health teams (Kurtz, Thornes & Wolkind 1994). There was then pressure on social workers to give priority to child protection issues, so that they were either removed from the multidisciplinary teams, or were less available as therapists. New outpatient services were established, although the size and staffing depended on local pressures and personalities rather than population need. Some smaller residential units were closed, as they were not thought to be economic, and separating younger children from their families for residential treatment was used only when other therapies had been tried.

Child psychiatry was a small specialty, which received little government attention for many years. Waiting lists began to mount as other agencies that had provided support to families changed the focus of their work. Social workers were no longer in a position to offer ongoing therapeutic work, as there was a greater emphasis given to child protection and formal assessment (Health Advisory Service 1995). Schools became under pressure to increase the academic success of the students and so the needs of the curriculum had to be given priority over pastoral work. More children were excluded from school either temporarily or permanently. This resulted in many child psychiatry services having an increase of referrals which led to waiting lists of months, if not years.

NEW DEVELOPMENTS IN CAMHS IN BRITAIN

In 1995 the NHS Health Advisory Service published a thematic review entitled *Together We Stand – The Commissioning, Role and Management of Child and Adolescent Mental Health Services*. The overall mental health needs of all children were considered and an acknowledgement was made of the contribution of all agencies in promoting this. The Department of Health (1995) adopted a similar approach in *A Handbook on Child and Adolescent Mental Health*.

These key documents described a four-tiered model of service delivery (Table 1.1), and Kurtz (1996) suggested Health Promotion as an additional tier. The tiers described in *Together We Stand* incorporated all the agencies and professions associated with the delivery of CAMHS. Occupational therapists were included, although they were added only shortly before publication as a result of the intervention of the occupational therapist at the Department of Health.

New government funding became available for CAMHS in the late 1990s and Health Commissioners are becoming more knowledgeable about these services. There is an attempt to develop equitable services across the UK rather than the haphazard development seen previously. Health authorities are establishing systems of joint agency planning to create local CAMH priorities.

THE TIERED APPROACH TO THE DELIVERY OF CAMHS

Health promotion

Families and social networks

The most important factor in the mental health of children is the nature of their care. Sensitive parents who are responsive to their children's needs and reciprocate their communications will aid the development of their children's psychological well-being. Families and social networks,

Table 1.1 Services offered in the tiered approach to child and adolescent mental health services

Tier	Function	Professionals/agencies
Health promotion	*Promotion of good parenting:* Parenting education in schools Contraceptive advice Antenatal education Postnatal support	Extended family and social network Personal and social education teachers School nurses Family planning advisers Midwives Health visitors
Tier 1: primary care	*Early intervention:* General advice on childcare/parenting Problem-solving approach Support in negotiating life events (e.g. bereavement, divorce) Early identification of mental health problems	Health visitors School nurses Social services Voluntary agencies Teachers Educational welfare officers
Filter between Tiers 1 and 2	Mapping of services Consultation Assessment	Primary mental health worker
Tier 2a: network of professionals working independently	*Community base:* Identification and treatment of mental disorder Training and consultation to professionals in Tier 1 Assessment for another tier Outreach work to families who are unwilling to use other services	Paediatricians Educational psychologists Clinical psychologists Child psychiatrists Paediatric occupational therapists
Tier 2b: multiagency teams	*Community base:* Mapping local services Training and consultation to professionals in Tier 1 Joint work with primary care professionals Outreach work to families Short-term direct work with families and children	Health service staff School nurses Psychiatric nurses Occupational therapists Clinical psychologists Social workers Teachers
Tier 3: specialist service – multidisciplinary team	*Child mental health clinic:* Assessment and treatment of child mental health disorders Assessment for referral to Tier 4 Contribution to training/consultation Tiers 1/2 Research and development	Child and adolescent psychiatrists Clinical psychologists Occupational therapists Psychiatric nurses Possibly: Social workers Teachers Child psychotherapists Art, music, drama therapists
Tier 4: tertiary services	*Supra-district provision:* Adolescent/children's inpatient units Secure forensic adolescent units Eating disorder units Specialist teams for sexual abuse or neuropsychiatric problems	As above

supporting parents in their role, also contribute to the mental health of children. Poverty, domestic violence and parental mental ill-health may make the task of parenting more difficult, and are known to be risk factors in the development of mental health problems in children.

Schools

An approach to education whereby children feel valued for their abilities leads to greater self-esteem. Systems in school that confront bullying and support children to overcome the effects of victimisation will also promote self-confidence. Personal and social education classes enable children to develop life skills that include social skills and childcare. Exclusion from school causes children to lose opportunities for the development of healthy peer group relationships and reduction of contact with adults who could be positive role models.

Tier 1: primary care

Recognition is now being given to the contribution made by primary care staff in the early intervention into children's mental health difficulties. Some 15% of children and young people may show mild emotional and behavioural problems (Kurtz 1996). Children or their families are more likely to seek advice from professionals they meet regularly either at school or at the health centre. This is seen as more readily available and less stigmatising. There is an opportunity to address difficulties much earlier if primary care workers are in a position to offer support. Children's normal responses to difficult life events such as bereavement or divorce could be supported by an early brief intervention. Some school nurses, health visitors and teachers are willing and able to support families through crises, but there are many other demands on their skills.

Tier 2: a community and multiagency approach

Some 7% of children will develop moderately severe mental health problems, which will need the attention of a professional experienced in this area (Kurtz 1996). Many of the developments over the years since the publication of the Health Advisory Service Review *Together We Stand* have taken place at this level. Not all areas have the network of independent professionals described in the review. Paediatricians and educational psychologists provide separate services, but in many localities clinical psychologists and psychiatrists work mainly within the Tier 3 multidisciplinary service, so there is little differentiation between Tier 2 and Tier 3.

The Health Advisory Service review suggested the creation of a new role, the primary mental health worker, whose function is to support and train the staff in Tier 1 and to act as a filter between Tiers 1 and 2. This is being interpreted and developed in varying ways across Britain (Primary Mental Health Workers Conference Report 1999). It has also coincided with increased government funding for CAMHS such as the Mental Health Specific Grant, now the Mental Health Grant, the Modernisation Funds and Waiting List Initiative funding. Primary mental health workers may be appointed to cover a specific geographical area, such as a Primary Care Group boundary or area of specific need as in Youth Offender Teams. Other posts are jointly commissioned by health and social service departments, for instance to support the needs of children in the care of the local authority, whilst others are existing members of a Tier 3 service with an additional responsibility. Some primary mental health workers are linked to or placed within a Tier 3 service and so are able to liaise between the multidisciplinary teams and other agencies. In other areas social service departments employ a small team of workers with backgrounds in health, social services and education (Gregory 1998).

The role of primary mental health workers encompasses the following:

- mapping of existing contributions to CAMHS
- advice on referral routes
- training of and consultation with Tier 1 staff
- working with the systems surrounding a child and family
- advice/consultation to families
- short-term direct work with children and families where there are emerging mental health difficulties
- referral to Tier 3 multidisciplinary services.

Primary mental health workers have professional backgrounds in health (school nurses, psychiatric nurses, occupational therapists), social services and education. Occupational therapists may use their experience in assessing the child in all aspects of life invaluable, although some may find that there is insufficient direct work to utilise all their skills. Where small teams (Gregory 1998) develop, an occupational therapist may find more opportunities to use therapeutic approaches. There is, however, the opportunity to develop the potential of occupational therapy to be a health-promoting profession, based on the occupational perspective of health developed by Wilcock. This will be developed further in Chapter 2.

Tier 3: a multidisciplinary service

Multidisciplinary outpatient teams provide a service to children, adolescents and their families to assess and treat CAMH disorders. Some 1.85% of children are said to experience the severe and complex problems that require intervention at this level (Kurtz 1996). The teams vary in size and in the range of professionals included. Most consist of child psychiatrists and at least one other profession, frequently psychiatric nurses or social workers (Audit Commission 1999). Some professionals provide services at both Tiers 2 and 3. Clinical psychologists may be members of the multidisciplinary team and/or function separately as a psychology department. There are a growing number of occupational therapists working in these teams. In 1984, Jeffrey, Lyne & Redfern found 10 child psychiatry outpatient services employing occupational therapists. More Tier 3 services try to recruit occupational therapists but find it difficult to recruit staff to single-handed posts, as there is a lack of experienced therapists in this field. In some areas, paediatric occupational therapists are asked to provide a service to CAMH teams. The Audit Commission (1999) found that occupational therapists represented 4% of the personnel providing CAMHS.

Tier 4: tertiary services

These are the more specialised services, often offering regional residential units for children or adolescents. They may specialise in a particular

area such as eating disorders or forensic psychiatry. Only 0.075% children are thought to require this level of intervention (Kurtz 1996). Jeffrey identified occupational therapists working in 45 Day or Residential facilities (Jeffrey, Lyne & Redfern 1984). Kurtz, Thornes & Wolkind (1994) found that two-thirds of inpatient units had occupational therapists. The reduction in number of inpatient units may have affected this group of therapists, although some have transferred to outpatient services.

It is important to understand the changes taking place in the late 1990s in order to ensure that health commissioners and managers begin to be aware of the profession's contribution to these developments. New areas of work with children and adolescents are being created with the following programmes, all of which are multi-agency initiatives and represent a new way of configuring services:

• Sure Start – aimed at supporting families with preschool children in order to prevent problems developing (Department of Education and Employment 1999).
• Youth Offender Teams – multiagency teams aimed at reducing youth offending by a variety of interventions and preventive work (Crime and Disorder Act 1998).
• Looked After Children initiatives – groups of children with major mental health needs who in the past have not always had access to treatment (Department of Health 1999).

SUMMARY OF THE ROLE OF OCCUPATIONAL THERAPISTS IN CAMHS

In 1984, Jeffrey, Lyne & Redfern located 82 occupational therapists working in the CAMH field; in 1999 the National Association of Paediatric Occupational Therapists (NAPOT) had approximately 100 members in CAMHS. There are a significant number of occupational therapists working in this field, particularly in adolescent mental health services, who are not members of NAPOT. Most occupational therapists are to be found in Tiers 3 and 4, but a growing number may take up posts in Tier 2 and in managing CAMHS.

Historically many occupational therapists have worked single handed (Jeffrey, Lyne & Redfern 1984) and have not had the advantage of peer professional support. Child and adolescent mental health services have been organised into multidisciplinary teams, where there has been considerable role blurring in order for a small group of staff to cover a range of interventions. Inevitably professional identity was compromised leading to a reduction in the available therapies. Lougher (1990) described the role of the occupational therapist as mainly using family therapy. Occupational therapy has been slower than other professions to develop a system of postgraduate education. There is growing interest in CAMHS shown by occupational therapists beginning to form regional networks within NAPOT or requesting status as a Special Interest Group within the College of Occupational Therapists. Chapter 2 looks in more detail at the developing role of occupational therapy in CAMHS.

REFERENCES

Audit Commission 1999 National report: children in mind – child and adolescent mental health services. HMSO, London
Creek J (ed) 1997 Occupational therapy and mental health. Churchill Livingstone, Edinburgh
Crime and Disorder Act 1998 (Youth Offending Teams, Section 39, Part III). HMSO, London
Department of Education and Employment 1999 Sure Start – making a difference for children and families. DfEE Publications, London
Department of Health 1999 Working together to safeguard children. DoH Publications, London
Department of Health and Department for Education 1995 A handbook on child and adolescent mental health. HMSO, Manchester
Graham P J 1994 Paediatrics and child psychiatry: past, present and future. Acta Paedatrica 83(8):880–883
Gregory D 1998 The family support team – CAMH project developing Tier 2 Services in Norfolk. Norfolk Social Services Department, Norwich
Health Advisory Service 1995 Together we stand – the commissioning, role and management of child and adolescent mental health services. HMSO, London
Jeffrey L, Lyne S, Redfern F 1984 Child and adolescent psychiatry – survey 1984. British Journal of Occupational Therapy 47(12):370–372
Kurtz Z 1996 Treating children well: a guide to using the evidence base in commissioning and managing services for the mental health of children and young people. The Mental Health Foundation, London
Kurtz Z, Thornes R, Wolkind S 1994 Services for the mental health of children and young people in England: a national review. Report to the Department of Health. South West Thames Regional Health Authority, London
Lougher L 1990 Child and family. In: Creek J (ed) Occupational therapy and mental health. Churchill Livingstone, Edinburgh, ch. 22, p 371
Parry Jones W 1989 The history of child and adolescent psychiatry: its present day relevance. Journal of Child Psychology and Psychiatry 30(1):3–11
Primary Mental Health Workers First Conference Report 1999 Held at NSPCC Conference Centre, Leicester. Child & Adolescent Mental Health Service, Leicester
Rockey J 1987 Occupational therapy with children. British Journal of Occupational Therapy 50(10):341–342
Sayers J 1991 Mothering psychoanalysis. Penguin Books, London
Wilcock A 1998 An occupational perspective of health. Slack, Thorofare, New Jersey

FURTHER READING

Audit Commission 1999 National report: children in mind – child and adolescent mental health services. HMSO, London

Health Advisory Service 1995 Together we stand – the commissioning, role and management of child and adolescent mental health services. HMSO, London

USEFUL ADDRESSES

National Association of Paediatric Occupational Therapists (NAPOT)

65 Prestbury Road
Wilmslow SK9 2LL, UK
(publishes three journals per year)

Association for Child Psychology and Psychiatry (ACPP)

St Saviour's House,
39–41 Union Street,
London SE1 1SD, UK

(publishes *The Journal of Child Psychology and Psychiatry*, *Child Psychology* and *Psychiatry Review*)

Young Minds

102–108 Clerkenwell Road,
London EC1M 5SA, UK
(publishes a magazine every 2 months which covers news on issues affecting children's emotional and mental health)

2

Occupational therapy in child and adolescent mental health services

Lesley Lougher

CHAPTER CONTENTS

INTRODUCTION

The aim of this chapter is to examine the position of occupational therapists in child and adolescent mental health services (CAMHS). Most will be working in teams providing a service at Tier 2/3 level or residential units at Tier 4 (Health Advisory Service 1995). In Britain most therapists are working in multidisciplinary teams, many single-handed therapists making little contact with others in their profession. In order to develop further skills and deepen their understanding, they often take postgraduate courses in specific areas of treatment such as play therapy, family therapy or other types of psychotherapy. Unlike nursing, which has had an accredited system of postgraduate study for over 30 years, occupational therapy has only relatively recently begun to establish Masters' degrees. Access to these courses still incurs a considerable degree of personal commitment as they may not be available from the local health services training consortia. A nurse may have the opportunity to take up a modular Master's degree, taught near to the place of work and with CAMHS units available. Some of these courses are now being made available to other disciplines but, with one notable exception, this is a recent phenomenon.

Occupational therapists graduating in Britain before the early 1990s did not have a firm understanding of models and theories of occupational therapy. Particularly in psychiatry, occupational therapists struggled to explain the uniqueness of their contribution and, without access to further education, gave up the struggle opting instead for other therapeutic approaches in which to demonstrate their developing expertise. This has been particularly true in CAMHS, where an occupational therapist was more likely to be the only member of the profession in a multidisciplinary team. Many of the following chapters demonstrate how a generation of therapists had to gain training from outside the profession to raise their level of practice and theoretical understanding to a postgraduate level. The contributors here have used the training to augment their occupational therapy practice; others have left to pursue other careers.

Health service professions such as nursing and occupational therapy were established as mainly women's professions, with a flattened career structure created for women who may leave when they have children or who work as part-timers. This no longer represents the career path of many women who choose not to have children or who are lone parents or main wage earner. Nursing, perhaps owing to the size of the profession or greater numbers of men, has more scope for advancement, although this may lead out of the clinical field into management. An occupational therapist in Britain could reach a Head 3 post within 9 years of qualification, possibly much sooner. Where is she to go then for the next

40 years of her professional life? This is not only a problem for occupational therapists in CAMHS, but may be more critical because of the scarcity of Head Occupational Therapist posts. Postgraduate education will not necessarily result in promotion, nor is experience and expertise being recognised financially.

Notwithstanding, a number of occupational therapists have worked in CAMHS for many years. They are not always identified as occupational therapists and yet their work certainly is occupational therapy. Few write about what they do, although many can be found lecturing at conferences, running workshops and seminars. Most are highly valued within their teams, although only recently has this regard begun to encompass the profession rather than the individual.

THE INVISIBLE PROFESSION?

Some occupational therapists in Britain and the USA have been writing about their work in CAMHS in the occupational therapy publications since the 1950s (Rockey 1987). Occupational therapy textbooks have also included references to work with children and adolescents with mental health problems (Creek 1990, 1997, Finlay 1997, Kielhofner 1995, Mosey 1973, 1986). One book has been co-authored by an occupational therapist (Kaplan & Telford 1998), giving an account of non-directive play therapy. There has been a steady flow of articles written for the occupational therapy press over the past 30 years (169 were identified between 1998 and 1970 on the OTDBase, Occupational Therapy Internet World); some of these will be considered below.

Little mention has been made of the profession in textbooks of child psychiatry. Rutter, Taylor & Hersov (1995) made no reference to occupational therapy; Lane & Miller (1992) made one; and Chesson & Chisolm (1996), exceptionally, allocated a chapter to the role of occupational therapy in child psychiatric units. Sholle-Martin & Alessi (1990) found few references in the US literature.

There are many possible reasons for this lack of recognition. Occupational therapy is a relatively small, mainly female, profession. There was a crisis in confidence within the profession 15–20 years ago, so that many of the senior practitioners now do not have the assurance of more recent graduates. These factors affect the whole profession but, perhaps of more significance in CAMHS, is the structure of the organisations. Whether delivering services at Tier 2, 3 or 4, a CAMH service in Britain usually consists of a small multidisciplinary team.

MULTIDISCIPLINARY TEAMS

Occupational therapists working in CAMHS have embraced the concept of the multidisciplinary team. This has been both a source of support and of role confusion. CAMHS teams may be small so that a certain degree of role blurring is essential, but some occupational therapists have lost and even deny their professional identity, preferring to be described as play, family or child therapists according to their postgraduate training. This role doubt affected other professions such as doctors (Harrison 1989, Parry Jones 1989) at a time when the medical model of treatment was less prominent. This situation appears to be changing with the increasing use of medication for children's mental health disorders such as attention deficit/hyperactivity disorder (ADHD) and obsessive compulsive disorders.

Many writers from both CAMHS and adult mental health teams have struggled to define a multidisciplinary team. It may be described as no more than a group of professionals meeting regularly at a ward round (Cowan 1991). Steinberg (1986) suggested: 'the word team conveys the idea of unity in a common purpose, with individuality and individual action being subordinated to the beliefs and methods of the team, either by consensus or acceptance of the authority of the team's leader'. Parry Jones (1986) suggested a compromise between a traditional bureaucratic and an egalitarian structure. He described professions working together in a large multidisciplinary network, forming smaller, short-term teams to address a specific issue, either clinical or organisational. This would encourage disciplines to develop their particular skills rather than to blur roles for the sake of the team philosophy.

Struggles for team dominance may become crippling, leading some medical writers to propose the return to a consultant-led team (Mathai 1992, Silveira 1992). However, De Silva et al (1995) described a more peaceful process, emphasising that independent decision-making of team members, whilst sharing a common purpose, contributed to the shared knowledge from which therapeutic decisions result. They also suggested that other team members are not 'handmaidens of the doctors' and are to be treated on an equal professional footing.

None the less, Creek (1998), in her discussion of the difficulty occupational therapists experience in describing their work, has suggested that a predominantly female profession that is concerned with quality of life and enablement rather than cure struggles to find a common language with medical colleagues. She suggested that the 'opinion of a young female therapist is unlikely to be accorded equal respect with that of the more dominant, more senior or male members of the team. The doctor's truth is given more weight than the occupational therapist's truth' (Creek 1998, p. 130).

TASK OF THE CAMH MULTIDISCIPLINARY TEAM

There continues to be discussion as to the goals and tasks of the multidisciplinary team. These vary according to the setting: a ward-based team works with the same group of patients, each profession adding a different intervention. An outpatient team may work jointly with some families from referral, but a more common approach is for one professional to assess the family's needs and to call on other members of the team where their specific contribution may be helpful. Some services have a common assessment protocol but misunderstandings may arise where there is a lack of understanding about the type of assessments made by the professions. Doctors and occupational therapists are working from different frames of reference and models of treatment, so the content and purpose of the assessments may not be interchangeable. Ambelas (1991) wrote about the task of treatment

Table 2.1   Tasks of the multidisciplinary team

	Processes		
Tasks	Information gathering	Assessment	Outcome
Case management	From social network: family, school and other agencies	Of overall needs	Social or therapeutic intervention
Diagnosis	Medical investigations Formal assessments: psychometric, occupational therapy	Formulation of diagnosis	Prescription of treatment
Therapy	As to suitability for treatment	Treatment plan	Application of therapeutic technique

of the multidisciplinary team and separated case management assessment from assessment for therapy. Meeson (1998) discussed the role of care management and the importance of assessing the individual's overall needs in occupational therapy practice.

Table 2.1 shows three aspects of treatment, each having similar stages and terminology but actually seeking to achieve a different outcome. Occupational therapists may take responsibility for Case Management and Therapeutic Intervention, and contribute to Diagnosis. There needs to be clarity as to the purpose of information gathering so that the most appropriate sources are approached. The content of an assessment should reflect the area of concern. Practitioners may confuse the task of assessing for treatment with that of assessing the overall needs of the child, which may also include decisions about involving other agencies and professions.

CORE SKILLS OF A PROFESSION

This leads to discussion of the professional core skills of team members. Joice & Coia (1989) used Ouvretveit's framework of four classes of skill to examine the role of occupational therapists in a multidisciplinary team. The first level of skill concerns the required clinical practices and procedures. Unlike other professions, there are no statutory requirements of occupational therapists. Social workers have obligations under the Children Act 1989 to assess children's needs for

protection, and both doctors and nurses have responsibilities under the Mental Health Act 1983. There are no restricted practices and procedures relating specifically to occupational therapy training. Some may suggest that formal assessment of functional capabilities in activities of daily living (ADL) should be made only by occupational therapists.

The second level of skill concerns the core skills of a profession. Joice & Coia (1989) suggest that individual professions should seek to describe only three or four core skills, and suggest the following for occupational therapy:

1. The use of selected activity, which has a purpose and meaning to the individual, as a treatment medium.
2. Activity analysis, which is the ability to break activities into physical, cognitive, interpersonal, social, behavioural and emotional demands made on patients and an understanding of how they may be used effectively to meet the needs of the individual.
3. Assessment and treatment of functional capabilities, which is the ability to assess and determine the extent to which a disturbance of mental state is affecting the functional capabilities of an individual, and the appropriate treatment for any problems identified.

Ouvretveit's third-level skills describe the core skills of a multidisciplinary team working in a specific field. In CAMHS, as well as adult mental health teams, these would include a basic knowledge of psychopathology, observation, counselling, education, research and management skills. There would also be common experience in groupwork skills and knowledge of different treatment approaches such as cognitive–behavioural, psychodynamic, medical, sociocultural and systems theory.

The fourth level of professional skills concerns the special skills and qualifications acquired through individual interest and enthusiasm. These require further training and supervision, and include play therapy, family therapy, gestalt therapy and psychodrama. Joice & Coia (1989, p. 467, my italics) warn:

A danger exists within the team (*or profession*) when professionals who acquire specialist skills prefer to practise these skills, neglecting their core skills or basic common skills, and can experience a resultant loss of identity.

This loss of identity has been an issue within CAMH teams where core skills have been devalued in the pursuit of a common ideology such as family therapy. This is no longer acceptable as users and commissioners of healthcare services demand a range of treatment options to meet their needs and preferences. All professions have had to re-examine their core skills in order to justify their place within the team. Small teams in areas where recruitment is difficult may advertise for applicants from a range of professional backgrounds for one post. The third and fourth levels of skills of the successful candidate may be similar, but the service will also gain from a variety of second-level skills.

Definitions of occupational therapy abound, but Creek's description of the occupational therapy approach is perhaps most pertinent to therapists working in CAMHS:

The uniqueness of the occupational therapy approach to psychosocial dysfunction lies in the philosophy of human beings having the ability to influence their own health through occupation. (Creek 1997, p. 32)

This suggests a wider view of occupational therapy than that proposed by Joice & Coia (1989), and is supported by Olson (see Ch. 12), who warns against the profession focusing only on the performance components of occupation.

OCCUPATIONAL THERAPY IN CAMHS LITERATURE

Within this book, a greater confidence in the unique contribution of occupational therapy to this field of practice can be found in the chapters written by authors from the United States and New Zealand. In order to discover how occupational therapists define their work in CAMHS, a comparison of a selection of papers written by occupational therapists in Britain, United States and Canada was made.

Occupational therapy in CAMHS is not represented widely in the literature of any of the three countries. There appear to be keynote articles, which are quoted by other authors as being significant in the development of therapeutic approaches in this area of practice. A comparison of these shows the strengths and shortfalls in the development of occupational therapy practice in CAMHS.

British Journal of Occupational Therapy

A review of articles published since the 1970s demonstrates a noticeable trend in the development of occupational therapy in this field of practice. Most contributions describe a specific therapeutic intervention, technique or case history with very little discussion of theoretical approach and sparse evidence of research. Many of the papers that are exceptions to this rule are written by a series of occupational therapists employed in one unit over a period of 30 years, now known as the Fleming Nuffield Unit for Children and Young People in Newcastle. It is perhaps no coincidence that occupational therapists employed there have had access to postgraduate education in CAMHS over this period of time (Ackral, Kolvin & Scott 1968).

The papers selected here are concerned predominantly with the therapeutic use of play. There are many other articles published describing group work, using social skills or psychodynamic approaches, but they tend towards being informative rather than adding to occupational therapy theory, and so were not selected for the present discussion. This does result in a bias towards occupational therapy used with children rather than adolescents. It could be suggested that many therapists working with adolescents perceive their role more in terms of being generic members of multidisciplinary teams, than in seeking to develop a specifically occupational therapy approach to working with young people.

In 1973 Widdup and Jeffrey started publishing articles in the Journal. Widdup (1973) described the staffing and facilities required to set up an occupational therapy department within a child psychiatry unit. She also began a discussion on the therapeutic values of different forms of play: developmental, creative and expressive, fantasy and social play, as well as the use of activities. This was a theme developed by Lily Jeffrey, who became the main exponent of the role of occupational therapists in CAMHS in Britain over the following 20 years. Her fellowship thesis in 1981 was entitled: 'Exploration of the use of therapeutic play in the rehabilitation of psychologically disturbed children' (Jeffrey 1981). She presented ideas for the development of the profession in this area, identifying the need for postregistration studies and research, and describing the therapeutic processes of occupational therapy in this field as:

1. The child's relationship with the occupational therapist in individual therapy
2. The use of the child's peer group in group therapy
3. The child's participation in the activity i.e. Therapeutic Play, which is the treatment medium
4. The child's intrapsychic response to the three previous factors (Jeffrey 1982, p. 331)

There then followed a survey of the extent of occupational therapy services in child psychiatry (Jeffrey, Lyne & Fedfern 1984) (see Ch. 1). Jeffrey's contribution to the profession's body of knowledge was in her presentation of the model for play therapy using developmental theories, described as Developmental Play Therapy (Jeffrey 1984). This model provides a method of assessing the child's level of development and a technique for enabling the therapist to provide the therapeutic experience necessary to further growth. It is also a tool for measuring progress and was used by Bell, Lyne & Kolvin (1989) in

their research into a method of intervention in, and prevention of the effects of, multiple deprivation on inner-city infant schoolchildren. They were able to demonstrate some immediate effects in the increase in creative play and decrease in aggressive and regressive play. Longer-term outcomes were still awaited. Jeffrey has continued her promotion of developmental play therapy, even though she has moved into NHS management (Creek 1990, 1997, 1998).

In the 1990s Telford and Ainscough have continued the Fleming Nuffield contribution to the development of occupational therapy in child psychiatry in Britain. Their article concerning the combination of psychoanalytic insights with non-directive play therapy (Telford and Ainscough 1995) encouraged some debate within the profession, although none was submitted for publication. This was followed by a paper on the therapeutic value of activity in child psychiatry (Ainscough 1998), in which Ainscough described the use of activity as the 'third party' in the therapeutic relationship with children who find the lack of structure in non-directive play therapy too challenging. The approach is said to be of advantage to children diagnosed with conduct disorder, ADHD, learning difficulties and relationship/attachment disorders.

The Butterfly Children (Kaplan & Telford 1998) is the first book to be published on occupational therapy in CAMHS. It describes the treatment of a 7-year-old girl by an occupational therapist using non-directive play therapy. Valuable insights are also given into the work of the multidisciplinary team, showing the use of supervision, case reviews and cross-agency working.

Widdup, Jeffrey, Bell, Lyne, Telford and Ainscough from Newcastle are not the only occupational therapists working in CAMHS who are developing approaches and ideas in therapy. Copley, Forryán & O'Neill (1987) from Birmingham have written about an approach to play therapy that uses concepts derived from psychoanalysis but draws a distinction between occupational therapy and intensive psychoanalytic work which requires further training and personal therapy. They suggest that an occupational therapist does not attempt to explore the child's inner world in depth, but uses an understanding of psychoanalytic theory 'to develop a receptiveness to a child's way of communicating his problems and anxieties' (Copley et al 1987, p. 413). Milston (1989, p. 437) described using 'a mix of cognitive-type therapy, reflection and psychodynamic technique' in which she also involved parents to develop the process of bonding and attachment where this had been problematic.

Milston (1989) acknowledged the support she received from her Head Occupational Therapist in being allowed monthly study time, which had enabled her to write the article. Perhaps this is a pointer as to why so few occupational therapists write for publication, although many are developing new therapeutic approaches, which they share readily. The annual conferences of the National Association of Paediatric Occupational Therapists have lectures, workshops and paper presentations by therapists working in this area. Many senior therapists, specialising in other treatment approaches such as play therapy or family therapy, may not be acknowledged as occupational therapists. It seems that, without the support and encouragement of postgraduate courses in occupational therapy and the availability of study time, this branch of the profession has mainly an oral tradition of passing on ideas and information. Hopefully the increasing requirement to demonstrate clinical effectiveness will support therapists in further study and publication.

Reade, Hunter & McMillan (1999) examined the effectiveness of play therapy with children who had experienced emotional deprivation. Reade found in her practice in child psychiatry that many children were referred with a range of problems, but that a common significant factor was the child's lack of basic care by nurturing parents. Occupational therapists in CAMHS use play therapeutically in the treatment of children; this process is frequently described as 'play therapy', whether or not the therapists have specific training in play therapy. Reade et al (1999) discussed the concept of emotional deprivation, the definitions of play therapy, and question the effectiveness of play therapy in the treatment of children who have been emotionally deprived.

They found a lack of outcome studies in the play therapy literature, and so examined the research into the effectiveness of child psychotherapy. Quantitative research studies show that behavioural approaches in therapy demonstrated more positive outcomes, possibly because specific behavioural changes were being measured, whereas the non-directive therapies were working towards less tangible outcomes. Target & Fonagy (1996) suggested that it was easier to demonstrate 'symptom change in more symptom focused therapies'. Reade et al (1999) reviewed case studies by occupational therapists (Jeffrey 1984, Milston 1989) in their examination of qualitative studies. They concluded (Reade et al 1999, p. 161) that occupational therapists 'should not be overwhelmed by their holistic philosophy' but should look to measure change within a specific piece of behaviour. They recommended use of the Canadian Occupational Performance Measure to provide a client-centred measure.

Examination of publications written by occupational therapists working in CAMHS in Britain over the past 30 years suggests that the dominant therapeutic approach is that of play therapy. Some authors have described a non-directive approach derived from Axline (Kaplan & Telford 1998), others a psychoanalytic influence (Copley, Forryan & O'Neill 1987), and some occupational therapists have developed their own models of practice (Jeffrey 1984, Milston 1989). Blunden (see Ch. 6) writes in more detail about the developments in play therapy and the theoretical models used by occupational therapists.

Occupational therapy in CAMHS in US and Canadian publications

The search for a role in child psychiatry

There is a greater tradition of research and publication amongst occupational therapists working in the USA, possibly as a result of greater access to postgraduate programmes of education. Notwithstanding this, one author was concerned that few articles had appeared in the previous 10 years written by occupational therapists working in the field of child psychiatry (Florey 1989).

Florey also found few references to occupational therapy in the child psychiatry textbooks. This field of practice was not claimed by either psychiatric or paediatric occupational therapists. Occupational therapists working with children were found to concentrate on sensorimotor development, with little mention of social and emotional development or the psychosocial components of performance.

Florey was concerned to encourage occupational therapists to take an interest in child psychiatry, so suggested four areas of knowledge needed by the entry-level therapist working with emotionally disturbed children:

- Human development throughout the life cycle, to include stages and tasks in sensory–motor, cognitive and social–emotional growth
- Purposeful activity in the areas of activities of daily living and specifically play
- Theoretical frameworks, in order to use appropriate occupational therapy frameworks for the specific client group
- Psychopathology – the problems and disorders commonly encountered in child psychiatry (Florey 1989, p. 367)

Florey suggested that paediatric occupational therapists, particularly those working in schools, should incorporate the treatment of children with emotional and behavioural problems into their practice. She was concerned that:

The pendulum of the paediatric knowledge base has swung entirely too far in the direction of neuromotor and sensory–motor concerns. It must swing back to include the social–emotional development and behaviour of children and adolescents. (Florey 1989, p. 368)

Sholle-Martin & Alessi (1990) sought to formulate a role for occupational therapy in child psychiatry, as they also found little reference to occupational therapy in the child psychiatry literature. They discovered more discussion of this area of practice in occupational therapy textbooks, although most focused on sensory integrative approaches. An exception was Cronin & Burnell (1989) who described practice based on psychoanalytic, social learning and behavioural, systems theory and developmental models as well as occupational therapy-based theories.

Sholle-Martin & Alessi (1990) suggested that occupational therapy in child psychiatry lacked delineation within the profession. They looked at the role of occupational therapists in the areas of diagnostic assessment, assessment and treatment strategies, and research.

Diagnostic assessment. They suggested that occupational therapy is able to contribute to the diagnostic assessment by the development of evaluation tools that measure key areas of competence and disability resulting from psychiatric disturbance in children.

Assessment and treatment strategies. Sholle-Martin & Alessi believe that occupational therapy practice needs to take a wider perspective than sensorimotor and neuromuscular skill needs. They propose the use of the Model of Human Occupation (Kielhofner 1995), as this provides a 'thorough assessment of the child's volitional, habituation, performance and environmental dimensions, could provide a view of his or her overall occupational functioning as well as a direction for treatment' (Sholle-Martin & Alessi 1990, p. 873). They direct particular attention to the examination of the organisation of occupational behaviours described as the 'habituation subsystem' in this model (p. 873):

the child's adaptive functioning is conceptualized as the organization of occupational behaviours (i.e. everyday self care, work and play activities) into patterns or routines that help to satisfy the child's need to explore and to be effective, as well as the demands of the environment.

Research. Sholle-Martin & Alessi found, at the time of their writing, that occupational therapy research in child psychiatry was 'virtually non-existent'. Some work had taken place on developing and using assessment and treatment planning based on the Model of Human Occupation (Sholle-Martin 1987).

Occupational behaviour frame of reference

There is an assumption that the adoption of an occupational therapy frame of reference enables the profession to develop and describe a unique role within the multidisciplinary team. Research into the effectiveness of interventions is therefore focused on those elements of change within a specific area of function, such as occupational behaviour. The British authors mentioned above do not explicitly use an occupational therapy frame of reference, although their practice may indicate awareness of the importance of occupational behaviour. The authors below use models developed from this framework, such as the Model of Human Occupation, in their practice in CAMHS.

Model of Human Occupation

Sholle-Martin (1987) described the application of the model by using human occupation assessment batteries on a short-term diagnostic and research unit for child and adolescent psychiatric inpatients. She also created a summary of occupational development in late childhood and adolescence (see Table 2.2), which is used to identify the components in the volitional, habituation and

performance subsystem. Sholle-Martin & Alessi (1990) found that the profile of adaptive functioning in a population of children hospitalised for psychiatric disturbances differed significantly from that of the normal standardised sample of the Vineland Adaptive Behavior Scales (VABS) (see Table 2.3). They concluded that the use of the VABS during hospitalisation provided a detailed baseline of adaptive functioning, a list of specific areas needing evaluation and change, and was useful in measuring treatment efficacy.

The Model of Human Occupation was also the theoretical framework used by Baron (1991) to design a treatment programme and assess its usefulness when working with a preschool child in an inpatient unit. A case history of a 4-year-old boy, Kevin, demonstrates how the four subsystems – volition, habituation, performance and environment – were used by the therapist to assess his general level of function. Baron also drew on Takata's four dimensions of milieu to nurture play (human, non-human, qualitative

Table 2.2 Summary of occupational development in late childhood and adolescence

	Late childhood	Adolescence
Volitional subsystem		
Personal causation	Develop a sense of competency Increase internal control	Maintain confidence Develop responsible self-determination
Values	Begin learning about values Develop awareness of future	Form a personal value system Anticipate success in adult roles
Interests	Develop interest patterns and increasingly differentiated and balanced interests	Develop new leisure interests and consider selection of a future vocation
Habituation subsystem		
Habits	Develop daily routines	Develop autonomy in regulating daily routines and work habits
Roles	Meet demands of new student role and increasing family responsibility Explore fantasised worker roles	Balance leisure and work roles Experiment with more adult roles
Performance subsystem		
Skills	Increase perceptual motor competency Increase reasoning and problem-solving skill Develop language, interaction skills and ability to follow rules	Adjust to rapid musculoskeletal growth and refine specific skills Increase cognitive ability, especially abstract thought Increase communication and interaction skills

From Sholle-Martin (1987) with permission from the American Occupational Therapy Association, Inc.

Table 2.3 Content description of the Vineland Adaptive Behavior Scales

Domain	Subdomain	Content
Communication	Receptive	Understanding of communication
	Expressive	Verbal expression
	Written	Reading and writing
Daily living skills	Personal	Self-care (e.g. dressing, eating, hygiene)
	Domestic	Performance of household tasks
	Community	Use of time, money, telephone and job skills
Socialisation	Interpersonal relationships	Interaction with others
	Play and leisure time	Performance in play and use of leisure time
	Coping skills	Responsibility and sensitivity to others
Motor skills	Gross	Use of arms and legs for movement and coordination
	Fine	Use of hands and fingers for object manipulation

From Sholle-Martin & Alessi (1990), who cite Sparrow S S, Balla D A and Cicchetti D V 1985 Vineland Adaptive Behavior Scales (classroom edition) with permission from the American Occupational Therapy Association, Inc. American Guidance Service, Circle Pines, MN.

and quantative aspects) in order to design an event she named a Playfair. This incorporated four activities – bowling, story corner, art and snacks – with opportunities to practise taking turns, sharing, organising and having fun. Baron (1991, p. 54) summarises the outcome thus:

During the Playfair, he engaged in numerous mastery experiences, each fostering enjoyment and motivation to move fluidly from activity. As he experienced his skills as strengths and not as limitations, it offered him a different kind of feedback about himself as a player, friend and child-interacting-with-caregiver. He also experienced himself interacting with a safe, trusting and nurturing environment. This multitude of experiences freed him to play in a more competent, satisfying, magical way.

This use of a model has enabled Baron to give a more detailed evaluation along several parameters. Other occupational therapists may well achieve the same outcome from similar activities, but may have had difficulties in defining the changes in Kevin's behaviour.

Two interventions for Attention Deficit/Hyperactivity Disorder

This disorder has received more notice in Britain in the late 1990s. Ainscough (1998) refered to the value of an activities based approach in the treat-

ment of these children. The OTDBASE lists 20 articles written between 1972 and 1998 by occupational therapists working with children suffering from ADHD. The main clinically effective treatment for this condition is stimulant medication, usually methylphenidate, commonly known as Ritalin. This is a short-acting medication and is given to the children whilst they are at school in order to control hyperactivity, impulsivity and inattention. It is not usually used whilst the child is at home so there is still a need to look at other methods of managing the difficulties, which may have detrimental effects on family life and the child's social development. This is a disorder where a focus on occupational behaviour with particular emphasis on the habituation subsystem is required. The establishment of clear routines in the family is essential and the child needs to develop strategies in order to gain control over impulsiveness and inattention. Two papers have been selected for discussion here, as they use an occupational behaviour frame of reference in treating the child (Kwako 1981) and the family (Segal 1998).

Kwako studied the effectiveness of a relaxation therapy programme with a sample of 16 hyperactive and learning disabled boys. The author aimed to discover an alternative or additional intervention to the prescription of stimulant medication, in order to change the established negative patterns and to prevent developmental dysfunction. Relaxation techniques could be used effectively by parents, teachers and clinicians, and as a method of self-regulation for the children. Kwako suggested that competence in the ability to use methods of relaxation increases the potential to achieve self-mastery. She used the Jacobson system of progressive relaxation in therapy and devised a battery of tests to assess motor, visual, behavioural and psychological changes. The addition of regular intervals of relaxation therapy was shown to be an essential component of the development of self-regulatory skills for this client group due to the significant improvements in attention span and impulsivity.

Segal (1998) also agrees that ADHD is a disorder that may reduce the child's achievement of occupational competence. The purpose of her study was 'to understand the daily experiences of families with children who have ADHD and how they adapt their daily routines to enable their children's occupational competence' (p. 287). The most difficult times of the day identified by the families were found to be the morning before school and the evening homework sessions. All developed strategies to enable the child's occupational competence, but those families meeting with most success had adapted their own routines. Segal (1998, p. 291) suggested that occupational therapists discuss with the families the organisation of activities within the home and raise the following issues:

1. The other occupations that occur at home at the time when the suggested activity needs to be done.
2. The possibility of incorporating this activity whilst pursuing other occupations.
3. The possibility of rescheduling some of the occupations to another time or the possibility of getting help from another person.

This approach acknowledges that the management of the behaviour of a child with ADHD involves the whole family, as they reorganise their routines to enable the child to achieve greater competence in the achievement of routine tasks.

Occupational science: adolescent transition into adulthood programme

The first author writing about CAMHS interventions to cite the influence of the then emerging discipline of occupational science was Jeanne Jackson from the University of Southern California (Jackson 1990). Her programme was designed for adolescents with a variety of physical, emotional or communication learning disabilities, to facilitate their transition from adolescent to adult roles. Students were encouraged and supported to try out new experiences, to take risks and to learn how to problem-solve. By recognising their abilities and strengths, they could then exercise choice in developing goals for the future. Jackson drew on Reilly's work in building a philosophy for occupational therapy. She selected four of Reilly's 'conceptual threads' – occupations and occupational role, environment, independence and adaptation – as having specific relevance to the design of the Independent Living Skills Transition Program.

Occupations and occupational role. Occupations were described as vehicles through which satisfaction could be experienced in day-to-day existence and that also provided opportunities for risk-taking, problem-solving as well as pleasure in achievement. Occupational role acquisition was seen as evolving throughout the lifespan: from the preschool child, through schoolchild, student, worker, parent and retired person roles. 'Thus, the rules, skills and habits acquired during childhood play lay the foundation for the study habits and personal interaction skills of the adolescent which again mature and evolve into the job skills and work habits of the adult' (Jackson 1990, p. 35). Adolescence is a period of role transition, where future possibilities are explored in fantasy: shall I be a model, a firefighter or perhaps a teacher? This is followed by more realistic assessments of capabilities to direct choice towards more achievable goals, which is particularly important for the young people on Jackson's programme, who had specific disabilities to take into consideration.

Environment. This includes the therapeutic milieu, which needs to allow opportunities for decision-making and problem-solving, and to provide a sufficient degree of challenge to match the individual's skills. It is also suggested that the occupational therapy environment should encompass the day-to-day realities of home, school and work. Jackson draws on the theory of locus of control to explain an individual's relationship to their environment. Some individuals are described as having an internal locus of control, whereby they face the challenges of life with some optimism, believing they are able to influence their environment. Those said to have an external locus of control perceive obstacles set to frustrate them over which they have little power.

Independence. Jackson suggests there are two personal components to independence: competence and autonomy.

Competence refers to the patient's ability to use his or her physical, emotional and cognitive resources to choose an appropriate course of action in effectively interacting with his or her physical, social and personal environment. It is acquired through a process of becoming in touch with one's desires, choosing a plan of action to satisfy those desires, implementing the plan and evaluating outcomes.

Autonomy… includes the freedom to choose and regulate one's own lifestyle and prioritize activities according to one's own interests and values. It… demands accuracy in self appraisal, risk taking and a self perception which considers residual abilities rather than disability. (Jackson 1990, p. 38)

Adaptation. Jackson draws on research from social psychology on the subjective responses of adolescents to their daily activity patterns. It was found that they fluctuated between boredom and excitement, perceiving their occupations as either overwhelming and therefore stress-provoking, or underchallenging leading to boredom. Adolescents did not have a clear perception of their abilities, were unable to structure their environment or set meaningful goals. There were times, however, when they experienced a balance between the demands of the activity and their skills. This was described as a 'flow experience', characterised by the subjective experience of concentration, a loss of

self, a set of rules and a clear expectation of outcome. A key task of adolescence is to learn how to develop more complex patterns of behaviour to meet the increasing challenges of adulthood.

In using these four categories for the Independent Living Skills Transition Program, both the content and the environment were monitored. A centre was refurbished to provide living room, kitchen and office in which new skills could be practised. There was an expectation of active involvement, but there was also an acceptance of and willingness to work with the emotional extremes expressed by the students. The content of the programme included profiles of each student's pattern of daily activity, satisfaction with life, future aspirations, strategies in problem-solving and concept of self. A range of assessment tools was used to draw up the profiles. Students and therapists worked together to create individual programmes, designed to promote mastery in independent living skills and to develop coping strategies to deal with the challenges of adult life. The four areas addressed were leisure, prevocational, daily living and social communication skills.

Florey (1989) was concerned that, in the USA, occupational therapists had focused on the performance components to the exclusion of social and emotional development. In Britain the emphasis on play therapy suggests the dominance of the volitional subsystem as the area for intervention. Less attention is given specifically to the habituation subsystem and yet many of the children referred to CAMHS have not had the opportunity to develop regular routines and clear roles, given the multiple problems faced by their families.

SUMMARY OF THEORETICAL INFLUENCES

Occupational therapists use activities as a treatment medium to enable children to experience a sense of achievement, to learn new skills, to create a tangible representation of their experiences and feelings, or to learn how to work in partnership with others. This is a central part of the programme in residential and day units, and provides opportunities for assessment, either for diagnostic purposes or to measure the effectiveness of therapeutic interventions. Therapists working in outpatient services do not always have the same access to materials and ideal treatment environments, and so develop alternative ways of working. They may use treatment approaches derived from a variety of theoretical frameworks and wonder whether they are still practising occupational therapy.

In Britain, play therapy has been the treatment modality that seems to enhance occupational therapy with children, as it uses the major occupation of children to enable age-appropriate development or as a projective medium to work through trauma and loss. A systems approach such as family therapy is attractive to occupational therapists as it focuses on the context of the child's difficulties, so transferring them from a disorder of the individual to an imbalance in the system. Psychodynamic psychotherapy is used to understand the effect of early relationships on current difficulties. Interventions aimed at performance components such as sensory integrative therapy may be appropriate for some children where the lack of performance skills is the precursor or major factor in the disorder. However, for other children, such narrow focus may overlook difficulties in the family or wider context.

Occupational therapy practice in the field of child and adolescent mental health services has the opportunity to develop a treatment approach derived from the philosophy of occupational science. The family is the first source of role identity and provider of a structure of habits and routines from which the child develops skills and relationships. In a healthy family, the structure and routines are sufficiently flexible to respond to the differing needs of growing children. Preschool children require clear and consistent boundaries to protect and nurture them, whereas adolescents need more freedom to experiment and take risks in order to learn by their mistakes. The transition points may be used to re-examine roles, to make changes in routines and to recontract the family's relationship to the wider society. These routines are made up of a network of occupations, some of which may be in a state of tension. A mother in paid employment has to balance the occupation of working with that of giving care to her children. Parents of a new baby not only have to add the roles of mother and father to that of partners, but find that looking after the baby may become the dominant occupation. For new parents, leisure interests, household tasks and even personal care have to be fitted into the times when the baby sleeps.

The content of an occupational therapy session in a CAMH outpatient service may not include participation in a practical activity, but intervention is focused on the changing roles, the balance of occupations and the family's use of the environment. Many of the children referred to CAMHS live in families experiencing multiple problems. Parents may be struggling with poverty, poor housing, mental health problems, substance misuse, relationship problems and marital breakdown, all factors that have an impact on the children. Some families manage adversity in a manner that does not further handicap their children. A smooth-running household, where meals are produced when expected, a reasonable standard of cleanliness is maintained and there are routines for getting up, going to and from school, and going to bed, will enable the child to make use of other opportunities. Parents of very young children may struggle with their new roles and balance of occupations and so fail to create clear routines for the family. Discussion of parenting skills requires more than advice on child discipline and information on child development. Attachment relationships are formed in the context of activities, be it feeding, bathing or playing. Olson (see Ch. 12) discusses activity programmes involving parents and children.

Occupational therapists working in CAMHS have the opportunity to use the knowledge of the value of occupations in promoting the mental health of children, within the tiered system of service delivery advocated by the NHS Health Advisory Service review (1995). In Tier 4 services, usually residential or day treatment centres, the main focus of treatment is on the individual child, with some involvement of the carers. The child's occupational performance is central to the treatment, whether in ADL or specific therapeutic programmes. Occupational therapists working in a Tier 3 service will use therapeutic approaches, derived from a variety of theoretical frameworks, but will have greater access to the child's role in the community. (The tiers are not mutually exclusive and a therapist may work at several levels from the same organisation.)

Occupational therapy has established a role within Tiers 3 and 4, but new challenges lie ahead in the community approach. Ann Wilcock (1998, p. 344) believes the profession has a responsibility to share its knowledge more widely:

Health and wellbeing result from being in tune with our 'occupational' nature. For health and wellbeing to be experienced by individuals and communities, engagement in occupation needs to have meaning and be balanced between capacities, provide optimal opportunity for desired growth in individuals or groups, and be flexible enough to develop and change according to context and choice. Such engagement, if it is in accord with sociocultural values and the natural world, will enable individuals, families and communities to flourish. Rigorous exploration and sharing of this ideal, and taking action to ensure that it is considered wisely, could be our contribution to public health.

The increasing role of CAMHS in community health initiatives enables the development of interventions influenced by social, cultural and occupational perspectives of health. This creates opportunities for occupational therapy to contribute to the new approaches in the promotion of the mental health of children and families.

REFERENCES

Ackral M, Kolvin I, Scott D McL 1968 A post registration course in child psychiatry. Nursing Times, 5 April

Ainscough K 1998 The therapeutic value of activity in child psychiatry. British Journal of Occupational Therapy 61(5):223–226

Ambelas A 1991 The task of treatment and the multidisciplinary team. Psychiatric Bulletin 15:77–79

Baron K B 1991 The use of play in child psychiatry: reframing the therapeutic environment. Occupational Therapy in Mental Health 11:2–3

Bell V, Lyne S, Kolvin I 1989 Playgroup therapy with deprived children: community based early secondary prevention. British Journal of Occupational Therapy 52(12)

Chesson R, Chisholm D 1996 Child psychiatric units – at the crossroads. Jessica Kingsley, London

Copley B, Forryan B, O'Neill L 1987 Play therapy and counselling work with children. British Journal of Occupational Therapy 50(12):413–416

Cowan C 1991 Multidisciplinary involvement in hospital discharge. Psychiatric Bulletin 15(7)

Creek J (ed) 1990 Occupational therapy and mental health. Churchill Livingstone, Edinburgh

Creek J (ed) 1997 Occupational therapy and mental health, 2nd edn. Churchill Livingstone, Edinburgh

Creek J 1998 Communicating the nature and purpose of occupational therapy. In: Creek J (ed) 1998 Occupational therapy – new perspectives. Whurr, London, p 114

Cronin A F, Burnell D P 1989 Children with emotional or behavioural disorders. In: Pratt P N, Allen S A (eds) Occupational therapy for children, 2nd edn. Mosby, St Louis

De Silva P, Dodds P, Rainey J, Clayton J 1995 Management and the multidisciplinary team. In: Bhugra D, Burns A (eds) Management for psychiatrists, 2nd edn. Gaskell, London, p 121

Finlay L 1997 The practice of psychosocial occupational therapy, 2nd edn. Stanley Thornes, Cheltenham, UK

Florey L 1989 Treating the whole child: rhetoric or reality? American Journal of Occupational Therapy 43(6):365–369

Harrison T 1989 The role of the consultant psychiatrist in the clinical team. Psychiatric Bulletin 13(7)

Health Advisory Service 1995 Together we stand – the commissioning, role and management of child and adolescent mental health services. HMSO, London

Jackson J 1990 En route to adulthood: a high school transition program for adolescents with disabilities. In: Johnson J, Yerxa E (eds) Occupational science – the foundation for new models of practice. Haworth Press, New York, p 33

Jeffrey L 1973 Child psychiatry – the need for occupational therapy. British Journal of Occupational Therapy 36(8):429–437

Jeffrey L 1981 Explorations of the use of therapeutic play in the rehabilitation of psychologically disturbed children. Fellowship thesis. College of Occupational Therapists, London

Jeffrey L 1982 Occupational therapy in child and adolescent psychiatry – the future. British Journal of Occupational Therapy 45(10):330–334

Jeffrey L 1984 Developmental play therapy: an assessment and therapeutic technique in child psychiatry. British Journal of Occupational Therapy 47(3):70–74

Jeffrey L, Lyne S, Redfern F 1984 Child and adolescent psychiatry – survey 1984. British Journal of Occupational Therapy 47(12):370–372

Joice A, Coia D 1989 A discussion on the skills of the occupational therapist working within a multidisciplinary team. British Journal of Occupational Therapy 52(12)

Kaplan C, Telford R 1998 The butterfly children – an account of non-directive play therapy. Churchill Livingstone

Kielhofner G 1995 A model of human occupation – theory and application, 2nd edn. Williams and Wilkins, Baltimore

Kwako R 1981 Relaxation as therapy for hyperactive children. Occupational Therapy in Mental Health 1(3):29–45

Lane D, Miller A (eds) 1992 Child and adolescent therapy. Open University, Buckingham, UK

Mathai J 1992 Equality in a child and adolescent psychiatry multidisciplinary team. Psychiatric Bulletin 16(1)

Meeson B 1998 Occupational therapy in community mental health. Part 1: Intervention choice. British Journal of Occupational Therapy 61(1):7–12

Milston A 1989 Establishing bonding: a case of rebirth? British Journal of Occupational Therapy 52(11):437–439

Mosey A C 1973 Activities therapy. Raven Press, New York

Mosey A C 1986 Psychosocial components of occupational therapy. Raven Press, New York

OTDBASE Source: http://www.mother.com/~ktherapy/ot

Parry Jones W L 1986 Multidisciplinary teamwork – help or hindrance? In: Steinberg D (ed) The adolescent unit – work and teamwork in adolescent psychiatry. John Wiley, Chichester, UK, p 193

Parry Jones W L 1989 The history of child and adolescent psychiatry: its present day relevance. Journal of Child Psychology and Psychiatry 30(1):3–11

Reade S, Hunter H, McMillan I 1999 Just playing… Is it time wasted? British Journal of Occupational Therapy 62(4):157–162

Rockey J 1987 Occupational therapy with children. British Journal of Occupational Therapy 50(10):341–342

Rutter M, Taylor E, Hersov L 1995 Child and adolescent psychiatry: modern approaches: Blackwell Science, Oxford

Segal R 1998 The construction of family occupations: a study of families with children who have attention deficit/hyperactivity disorder. Canadian Journal of Occupational Therapy 65(5):286–292

Sholle-Martin S 1987 Application of the Model of Human Occupation: assessment in child psychiatry. Occupational Therapy in Mental Health 7(2):3–22

Sholle-Martin S, Alessi N 1990 Formulating a role for occupational therapy in child psychiatry: a clinical application. American Journal of Occupational Therapy 44(10):871–882

Silveira W R 1992 Is there a case for unidisciplinary working in child psychiatry? Psychiatric Bulletin 16(1)

Steinberg D 1986 The adolescent unit-work and teamwork in adolescent psychiatry. John Wiley & Sons, Chichester

Target M, Fonagy P 1996 The psychological treatment of child and adolescent psychiatric disorders. In: Roth A, Fonagy P (eds) What works for whom? – a critical review of psychotherapy research. Guilford Press, New York

Telford R, Ainscough K 1995 Non-directive play therapy and psychodynamic theory: never the twain shall meet? British Journal of Occupational Therapy 58(5):201–203

Widdup J 1973 Occupational therapy staffing and facilities for a child psychiatry unit. British Journal of Occupational Therapy 36(8):438–446

Wilcock A 1998 Occupation for health. British Journal of Occupational Therapy 61(8):340–345

FURTHER READING

Creek J 2000 Occupational therapy and mental health, 3rd edn. Harcourt Publishers, Edinburgh (in press)

Kaplan C, Telford R 1998 The butterfly children – an account of non-directive play therapy. Churchill Livingstone, Edinburgh

Roth A, Fonagy P 1996 What works for whom? A critical review of psychotherapy research. Guilford Press, New York

Wilcock A 1998 An occupational perspective of health. Slack, Thorofare, New Jersey

3

Problems and disorders found in child and adolescent mental health

Alan Evans

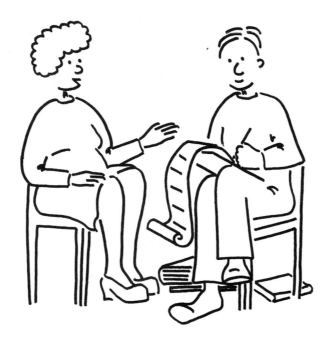

Occupational therapists working in child and adolescent mental health services require an understanding of the diagnostic categories used in child mental health. Irrespective of the model of practice adopted by the therapist, the medical model dominates in the area of problem diagnosis and so it is imperative that the process of diagnosis is understood by all members of the multidisciplinary team. It provides the common language and also a method of classifying and comparing groups of presenting features observed in a wide variety of differing clients. Without this ability it would be increasingly difficult to make decisions about possible treatment options and predictions of outcome.

First of all it is important to consider the reasons why children and adolescents present with a combination of symptoms, and why it is not appropriate to apply the knowledge of adult mental health as the only way to make sense of their presentation:

1. The child's symptoms must always be seen within a developmental framework. The presenting collections of features are in a constant state of change as the young person grows towards maturity.

2. The child is also developing within their environment, which will be significant to the manner in which the child adapts to the world around it. Any assessment must take into account the situation of the child, and the significant adults in the child's life, home and school situation. As the child develops towards adolescence, the networks become larger and the factors that influence the mental health of the child also increase.

CLASSIFICATION

The major systems of classifying mental health commonly used in Britain are the fourth edition of the *Diagnostic and Statistical Manual of Mental Disorders* (DSM-IV) and the International Classification of Disease-10 (ICD-10) for children and adolescents (World Health Organization 1992). The ICD-10 classification offers a multiaxial system, which takes into consideration other factors apart from the psychiatric syndrome; it also lists areas of specific developmental delay, the child's intellectual level, associated medical conditions and abnormal psychosocial circumstances. This

method of defining problems indicates the important contribution that all team members can make towards a more comprehensive assessment of a presenting child.

Wallace et al (1995) suggest that the difficulties that result in a referral to a child and adolescent mental health service constitutes the 'presenting problem', which may subsequently be addressed as the 'clinical problem' requiring intervention. The assessment will take into account 'severity', a multidimensional concept set against the following criteria (Wallace et al 1995):

- impairment – impact on individual, carer, environment
- age appropriateness – departure from expected developmental course or common patterns
- frequency
- duration
- persistence
- intensity
- extensiveness/pervasiveness
- intrusiveness
- manageability/controllability
- multiple presenting problems.

The assessment may result in a diagnosis of a disorder. Both problems and disorders may exist in the presence of risk factors, i.e. these may include children who have a history of offending, children in local authority care, children who have been sexually, physically or emotionally abused, or other significant factors.

This area is endless in scope and this chapter aims only to offer outlines of the most commonly seen conditions. The information will be presented in the following order:

1. Emotional disorders
2. Eating disorders
3. Conduct disorders
4. Hyperkinetic disorders
5. Developmental disorders.

EMOTIONAL DISORDERS

This range of conditions, often referred to as affective disorders, includes depression, anxiety, psychosomatic disorders, phobias, obsessional disorders, separation anxiety, school refusal, sibling rivalry, elective mutism, hysterical conversion, recurrent abdominal pain, suicide and self-harm.

Depression

Major depression in childhood is recognised by Wallace et al (1995) as occurring in 0.5–2.5% of children and 2–8% of adolescents. This covers a range of presentations from mild depression through to 'affective psychosis', where the depressive symptoms may be psychotic delusions or hallucinations. It has been recognised that the manner in which children present with depression differs from the presentation in adults, with the symptoms of the illness being masked and expressed through the development of phobias or delinquent behaviour. The depression may be secondary to other disorders, such as conduct disorder and school phobia, and may coexist with a range of physical conditions such as diabetes and epilepsy; it may also be a symptom of drug abuse.

The presentation of a depressed child includes a sad and low mood, a child lacking in motivation who has lost touch with previous interests, who has general low self-esteem and self-belief. Energy levels are often low and sleep may be disturbed. Suicidal thoughts may, in some cases, lead to suicide attempts. In adolescence attempted suicide has been found to be prevalent in 2–4% of young people, with actual suicide in 7.6 per 100 000 15–19 year olds. Depression in children and young people is often reactive to the environment, and it is important that any assessment of the child takes into account the full picture of the child's experience, calling on the resources of the whole treatment team.

Anxiety

The experience of some anxiety through childhood and into adolescence is inevitable. Anxiety is a normal reaction to the process of change and development that the child must negotiate. However, where the symptoms of anxiety begin to interfere with the child's ability to function competently in some aspects of life, treatment may need to be offered. Often children present with reactions to stressful situations such as separation anxiety, where the anxiety has not been negotiated but in some way avoided, leading to secondary symptoms such as school refusal or social isolation. The development of phobias in response to anxieties also serves as a method of avoidance. Children may also 'somatise' their anxiety: the worries may be expressed as physical complaints, such as stomach aches, sore throats and headaches.

It is also important to include panic disorder. Although this is relatively uncommon in children under 10 years of age, it has a prevalence rate in adolescents of between 0.6% and 5.4%. The development of panic attacks can be related to anxiety, and may be a symptom of an avoidance reaction such as school refusal or social avoidance.

Wallace et al (1995) gives the prevalence of emotional disorders with an onset in childhood as varying between 4.5% and 9.9% in inner-city areas. They add that emotional disorders account for 25–33% of all clinic attendances.

Obsessional disorders

These are conditions characterised by the presence of obsessional thoughts, which are intrusive in nature and which are maintained regardless of any evidence of their rationality. Obsessional thoughts may also be accompanied by compulsive actions, which result from the beliefs inherent in the thoughts, for example excessive hand-washing in a child, who is convinced of the need to protect themself from contamination. The child may develop complex patterns of ritualistic, repetitive behaviours, which are carried out as a result of 'magical' beliefs that the action will effect some control on life events. The obsessions and compulsions that accompany them are often unwelcome and distressing to the child.

Although many children develop some irrational thoughts and fears (e.g. not to walk on cracks in the pavement or the 'bogie man will get you'), it is when the symptoms begin to interfere with the child's daily functioning and quality of life that treatment is required. Obsessional behaviour is reported as rare in children, but increases in incidence in children from age 10 years upwards, being identified in 1.9% of adolescents.

EATING DISORDERS

In early childhood eating problems can revolve around the process of taking in food and nourishment. These may be seen as developmental tasks, which the child struggles to achieve. Appetite and feeding disturbances in young children are often symptomatic of a range of physical conditions; however, the emotional component of the disturbance in taking in nutrition from significant adults may also need to be considered. Food refusal can be an emotive subject within a family, and the focus of attention may need to be towards the quality of the parent–child relationship, especially if the child shows no sign of malnutrition. 'Pica', a condition where children eat items other than food, food refusal, faddiness, non-organic failure to thrive and obesity are all disorders that can present in childhood or adolescence.

Anorexia and anorexia nervosa

Anorexia relates to loss of appetite, which may be observed as a presenting symptom in a range of situations, for example as a side-effect of medication. The term is often used synonymously with anorexia nervosa, but the latter relates to a collection of symptoms that are characteristic of this condition.

Lask & Bryant-Waugh (1993) list the following features of the condition:

- Determined pursuit of thinness, through the reduction in food intake. This may be accompanied by a fear of obesity.
- Weight loss with failure to thrive. The authors point out that prepubescent children have very small fat deposits and therefore have little to lose before the weight loss causes concern.
- Refusal to take fluids can also increase the risk of dehydration.

- The patient with anorexia nervosa is often preoccupied with bodyweight and energy consumption, and knowledgeable about the calorific value of food items.
- Distorted body image is also common; sufferers are unable to question their belief that they are overweight, despite all evidence to the contrary.
- Self-induced vomiting is common in this presentation, as is excessive exercising. Sufferers may be engaging in exercise in the privacy of the bathroom or their own bedroom.
- Laxative abuse may also be employed in a minority of cases as a method of controlling weight, especially in older adolescents. The abuse of laxatives can lead to electrolyte and mineral deficiencies.
- Amenorrhoea occurs in girls, who have previously achieved this stage of development. When weight has fallen significantly, the menstrual cycle ceases; in most cases this resumes when appropriate bodyweight has been achieved.

Anorexia nervosa is identified in 0.5–1% of 12–19 year olds, and is noted to be eight to 12 times more common in girls than in boys.

Bulimia nervosa

Bulimia is also most common in adolescence, with the incidence peaking at about 19 years of age. The presentation is characterised by two criteria: an irresistible urge to eat followed by self-induced vomiting or purging, and a morbid fear of getting fat.

The typical pattern of eating of the bulimic patient is to take in large quantities of food very quickly, during which times the patient may report feeling out of control. The frequency of this bingeing behaviour may be between once a fortnight and four to five times a day. These binges may be preceded by feelings of low mood, loneliness or anxiety, and can last for between several minutes and a number of hours. Binge eating usually precedes vomiting, which may be self-induced, but in some cases is triggered by reflex action. The incidence of bulimia is estimated as 1.6–4% in adolescent girls and as 0.14–0.2% in adolescent boys.

CONDUCT DISORDERS

Conduct disorder consists of a collection of oppositional behaviours, often of an aggressive nature. The presenting child may have a single symptom or a collection of behaviours; these may consist of stealing, fire-setting, consistent aggressive behaviour at home or at school. The behaviour may be directed towards adults or other children. The setting for this behaviour may be relevant and helpful in assisting children and carers to make sense of the behaviour. Boys present more often than girls, at a ratio of 3:1. Cases where the patterns of repeated difficult behaviour are well established are the most resistant to change. Conduct disorders in childhood can place serious limitations on a child's ability to make and keep friendships. This consequently impacts on the young person's self-esteem and quality of life. Delayed development in the ability to function in a socially acceptable way may handicap the developing child up to and beyond their adolescence.

The behaviour may result in increasingly antisocial and even criminal activity: lying, stealing, truanting, aggressive behaviours, fire-setting, running away from home or violence. This behaviour may be part of a conduct disorder, but might also be due to a recognisable cause such as the child being bullied, or struggling with schoolwork that is beyond their ability.

HYPERKINETIC DISORDERS

Attention deficit/hyperactivity disorder (ADHD)

Children presenting with hyperactivity symptoms display an extensive inability to concentrate, alongside a general restlessness and distractibility, which can be seen to be of relatively long standing. This presentation may lead to the suspicion of a conduct disorder; however, now that the diagnosis of attention deficit disorder is gaining acceptance, a wider consensus exists about the criteria for diagnosis. Children with ADHD have an observable inability to take turns, to wait in line, to concentrate and to avoid being distracted. They may have delayed reading ability, have slowed development of speech, and find relationships difficult.

Wallace et al (1995) identified 1.7% of boys at primary school level displaying the condition, and noted that one in 200 in the whole population suffers from severe hyperkinetic disorders. The use of medication in these cases has been found to be helpful over the short term, often combined with behavioural or cognitive approaches.

DEVELOPMENTAL DISORDERS

Developmental disorders range from specific developmental delays in areas of speech and language, and motor development, through to the pervasive developmental delays of the autistic spectrum conditions, such as autism, Asperger syndrome and Rett syndrome.

Specific developmental delay

These conditions, such as abnormalities of speech and language development, and specific motor delay, may equally be presented to the paediatric services as to the mental health services, but can produce concern and distress within families. The development of language usage, recognition and articulation usually follows a similar progress over the first 5–7 years of a child's life. When this development is slower, the cause may be environmental or organic in origin. Accurate diagnosis of the stage in the language which is dysfunctional is vital to implementation of the correct treatment.

Pervasive developmental disorders

Infantile autism

Infantile autism is classified as a neurodevelopmental disorder, organic in nature, which affects a child's ability to process information cognitively and which inhibits the child's social functioning.

The incidence of the condition has been recognised as approximately four per 10 000 population, with a more common presentation in boys than in girls. For a diagnosis of infantile autism to be made, there needs to be evidence of delay or abnormal development within the first 3 years of life.

The presentation is signified by a number of developmental delays. These cover the range of areas from speech and language development through to behavioural and social limitations:

In the area of speech and communication, approximately half of children diagnosed lack any useful speech, and in cases where speech has developed there may be a lack of emotional expression, coupled with an inability to comprehend spoken language.

Socially the developing child will often have been described as passive and unresponsive; parents may describe their child as being resistant to being cuddled and showing little spontaneous affection. Normal separation anxiety may be lacking and the child may not display any joy at being reunited with a parent.

The developing child may show signs of behavioural abnormalities. With some evidence of repetitive behaviours and actions, these may include the preoccupation with objects or parts of objects, and possibly the development of routines that help to structure their daily tasks, with a marked inability to respond with flexibility.

Although most cases of early-onset autism are diagnosed in the first 3 years, some children move into middle childhood or adolescence before the condition is identified. Often this will be picked up at school. Asperger syndrome may be overlooked until later in a child's educational career owing to the normal development of speech and grammar associated with this condition.

Asperger syndrome

This condition is associated with autism in that much of the presentation is similar in nature. The incidence of Asperger syndrome is low (approximately 20 cases per 10 000 population) and its prevalence lies mainly in boys: only one in ten cases diagnosed are in girls.

Children present with difficulties in making or retaining relationships; they often find difficulty in extracting meaning from non-verbal cues. The sufferer may appear obstinate in manner and aggressive when asked to conform to other people's demands. Some children may present as clumsy and uncoordinated.

CONCLUSION

The disorders described here represent the most common or frequently discussed problems and disorders seen in child mental health Tier 3 services. Primary care workers, for example health visitors and school nurses, treat many of the emotional and behavioural problems experienced by children such as enuresis or sleep problems in young children.

A working knowledge of diagnostic categories is needed for occupational therapists in child and adolescent mental health services, but this method of describing problems by symptom does not describe the child's strengths or means of coping with adversity.

REFERENCES

Lask B, Bryant-Waugh R (eds) 1993 Childhood onset anorexia nervosa and related eating disorders. Lawrence Erlbaum, Hove, UK

Wallace SA, Crown JM, Berger M, Cox AD 1995 Epidemiologically based needs assessment; child and adolescent mental health. Published by NHS Executive.

World Health Organization 1992 International Classification of Disease (ICD 10). World Health Organization, Geneva

FURTHER READING

Barker P 1990 Basic child psychiatry. Blackwell Science, Oxford

Black D, Cottrell D 1993 Seminars in child and adolescent psychiatry. Royal College of Psychiatrists, London

Health Advisory Service 1995 Together we stand – the commissioning, role and management of child and adolescent mental health services. HMSO, London

Frames of reference used in CAMHS

SECTION CONTENTS

The frames of reference used by multidisciplinary teams in CAMHS are not always those encountered in undergraduate study by occupational therapists. In Chapter 4, Sue Pownall summarises the theories of child development commonly encountered, many of which may be familiar to occupational therapists. Attachment theory, described by Carol Hardy and Karin Prior in Chapter 5, underpins many of the problems experienced by children seen in CAMHS. Play is widely acknowledged as a treatment medium utilised by occupational therapists working with children, but the theories informing its use are not always fully understood. Pauline Blunden describes the therapeutic use of play in Chapter 6. Systems theory, introduced by Becky Durant in Chapter 7, enables the child to be understood within the context of the family and wider social network. Gita Ingram examines therapy employing a psychodynamic approach in Chapter 8. After reading this section, occupational therapists interested in working in CAMHS should have an awareness of the main theories informing practice in this area.

4

Aspects of child development

Sue Pownall

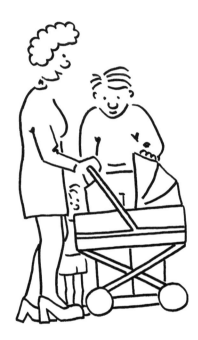

INTRODUCTION

There is a range of schools of thought on child and adolescent development, covering psycho-dynamic, cognitive and behavioural theories, and systemic models. It is also helpful to draw on child may be able to order objects on the basis of dimensions, such as height or weight. A 5-year-old may be able to go to a friend's house, but it is not until a few years later that they are able to draw a route map. The child is beginning to understand rules of cause and effect, and also moral rules, for example that spitting is wrong.

Piaget described the fourth stage of cognitive development as the formal operational stage; this occurs from around the age of 11 and 12 upwards. The child can think in abstract terms beyond experience. The adolescent is able to analyse and to plan for future possibilities. This stage is the transition to cognitive maturity.

Piaget and Inheldar stated that maturation of cognition is dependent on (Case-Smith, Allen & Nurse-Pratt 1996, p. 35):

1. Organic growth, especially maturation of the nervous system and endocrine glands.
2. Experience and the actions performed on objects.
3. Social interaction and transmissions.
4. A balance of opportunities for both assimilation and accommodation.

The significance of cognitive stages of development to the occupational therapist or other professionals working in child and adolescent mental health is to help them to understand the child's inner and outer world, and to relate to the child on his or her cognitive level and way of thinking. For the very young child a sensory approach may be useful. The assessment or treatment room or home may need to be a stimulating environment containing items with primary colours, textured materials and sounds. Toys that a baby can play with orally and simple musical instruments may be helpful. Occupational therapists, with their specialist approaches to activity, are ideally suited to working with young children. They may work jointly with the health visitor, who has a vital role to play.

In play therapy, the child may manifest their stage of cognitive development via play, making it essential for the occupational therapist to assess accurately whether the child is playing at a sensorimotor level or is using symbolic play in which feelings and thoughts are projected on to

toys. The child may be related to by story-telling. A range of therapeutic stories could be helpful as the child could learn through this medium. At the ages of 5–11 years the child may be able to write their own stories in sessions and understand more concepts. The older child will be able to grasp much more about the feelings of others, construction of events, thoughts and feelings about their own behaviour, and will develop much more insight. Poster work and group work are useful media. The occupational therapist therefore selects with the child activities adapted to suit the child's cognitive level. Special consideration should be given to the family's belief system and to aspects of learning difficulties, or to conditions such as ADHD. A surprising number of children can concentrate extremely well on a one to one basis. It is good to work with graded time-scales. Ten different activities may be needed to fill a 50-minute session in the first instance. The child should be rewarded at the end of each 5 minutes for concentration, and the occupational therapist can encourage the child or the parents to help increase the child's baseline ability.

The child may have learnt to feel very responsible for the world, for example for a death, a violent episode, a divorce or a separation. The professional working with the child needs to give careful and sensitive consideration to how the child is constructing their inner world. It may be useful for the professional to go on a counselling course, and to examine their own childhood.

ERIKSON'S STAGES OF PSYCHOSOCIAL DEVELOPMENT

Erik Erikson was born in Frankfurt in 1902. He was a friend of Freud. He was both a theologian and a poet and worked as a child counsellor, developing his psychosocial theory of development. His understanding was that the emergence of growth occurred as a consequence of psychosocial crises, i.e. that there was a tension between the competence of the child and the expectations of society. Development, he saw, was therefore a cog-wheeling motion between the individual and the environment, with each function of social development emerging in a systematic sequence appropriate for the developmental period. He believed that resolution of the tension resulted in the emergence of a virtue or strength.

Stage 1: Infancy (0–2 years)

Belief: I am what I am given.
Crisis: Trust versus mistrust. Trust – others are trustworthy and I will be taken care of. This means I am safe and I am okay. I am at peace and I fit in. Mistrust – others will not meet my needs and I am an alien, different not okay.

In this process, there needs to be an adequate matching between supply and the needs of the infant, together with the appropriate responses between mother and child. If the care-giver responds quickly in the early stages, the effect produced by the care-giver meeting the infant's needs is a belief that primal longings can be met, even when we are not being nice. The characteristic of this phase is a process of attachment to the care-giver.

A child's first cognitive development of logic is that when people or things are out of sight, they do not cease to exist. This provides the basis for a growing belief that the care-giver is always there, dependable and meeting the child's needs (object constancy). Out of this comes the deeper belief that mother is there for the child, no matter what the child does. The conviction is completed or fails by 36 months. There is increasing motor competence involving an ability to detach from the care-giver.

At this stage there is a belief in personal omnipotence. The child believes that they cause everything that happens in their world. This may give rise to the 'terrible 2s' stage. Experiences such as the death of a parent, or the father being violent towards the mother, may lead to an unresolved crisis in the young child. The implication is that the young child will form a social trust that their needs can be met, and this may lead to a self-trust, i.e. that the child does not have to earn approval but is acceptable as a human being. If this is not resolved, the child may go on in later life to a feeling of needing always to perform to earn approval from others in order to feel okay, a dissatisfaction with self, and possibly on to depressive episodes. The child needs a secure base to develop a sense of safety, secure love, and self-worth.

Stage 2: Toddlerhood (2–4 years)

Belief: I am what I will be.
Crisis: Autonomy versus shame or doubt.

Autonomy is a sense of being able to do something by yourself and to have control. Shame is a sense of not meeting up to expectations and being exposed as inferior. This feeling within a child may develop into anger and aggressiveness. The child may learn to doubt himself and his own competency.

The process by which autonomy occurs is by repetitive observation and practice. The care-givers are the role models and they also need to play a role in giving feedback to the toddler. The successful outcome of this process is a free will, a freedom to choose and that the choice was okay. The characteristics of this stage of development in a toddler's life are battles between the care-giver and the child for autonomy. The toddler undergoes toilet training. There is increasing separation from the care-giver in terms of distance and time, with the child returning to the care-giver frequently. There is a need for boundaries and a balance between rules and permissiveness. Enough freedom for the child suggests positive expectations of the child, whilst too much freedom brings the feeling of abandonment. Gender identity develops: 'boy versus girl'. There is a need to consider the impact of the single-parent female or male, and children being looked after by homosexual or lesbian couples, upon the child's gender identity. Also, due consideration needs to be paid to issues unique to the individual child such as disability, facial scarring through burns, sexual abuse, colour, children of mixed race parentage, immigrant children, children of different cultural and social backgrounds, and children from violent families.

Stage 3: Early school age (5–7 years)

Belief: I am what I imagine I can be.
Crisis: Initiative versus guilt.

may need help to construct a therapeutic story to change the ending of a bad dream to a good one. In case (3) it could be that a night-light needs to be left on, or the room decorated to help make it cosy or an object causing distress removed. In case (4) the child may need individual sessions to deal with post-traumatic stress.

The child and family's difficulties need careful screening by interview and taking a full history, to formulate a hypothesis about the aetiology of the difficulties, before deciding on the way forward and whether the child's development could be matured by using an approach based on the acquisitional theories. According to the cognitive viewpoint, a child learns by a process of memory storage and retrieval, and therefore a more comprehensive cognitive approach is necessary to tackle developmental difficulties.

SYSTEMS THEORY IN RELATION TO CHILD DEVELOPMENT

The child is reared within the context of caring adults and occupational therapists and other professionals therefore need to have some knowledge of systemic theories. In family therapy thinking, the child is viewed as a member of the family, acting and reacting with them. Structural family therapy was developed in the second half of the twentieth century. The child within the family environment does fit in with occupational therapy concepts; it may be that the problem does not lie solely within the child, but that the child is carrying the symptom for the family, and it is the family environment that needs to change. A child's behaviour may be triggered by the family context. Child-rearing offers many opportunities for individual growth and for strengthening the family system. At the same time, it is a field in which many fierce battles are fought, and unresolved conflicts of the spouses are often brought into the arena of child-rearing because the couple cannot separate parenting functions from spouse functions (Minuchin 1977).

What effect does family functioning have upon the child? What happens if one parent is strict and the other is lax? In the early process of social-isation, families mould and programme the child's behaviour and sense of identity. The sense of belonging comes with an accommodation on the child's part to family groups. Their sense of identity is influenced by a sense of belonging to a specific family. A sense of separateness and individuation occurs through participation within the family. When the child is born, the parental subsystem adapts from two people to three. As the child grows, developmental demands for autonomy and guidance impose demands on the parental subsystem. If the child is stressed, this can affect the relationship between the child and its parents, and also the parental relationships. The parents are expected to understand the developmental needs of the child. They need to nurture a young child, the amount depending on the child's developmental needs and the parents' capacity.

Effective child development occurs when both the child and parent accept the parent's authority. When the parents take up their responsibilities to formulate rules, this frees the child to grow and to develop autonomy. The parents can help the child to negotiate with them, even in a situation of unequal power. The parents can help a child with siblings, the skills of cooperation with siblings, competition, negotiation, and making friends. The family needs to adapt to the child's cognitive level and belief systems.

Family dysfunction can affect all members. There is a need for the occupational therapist to help the family to consider the needs of the siblings of children with difficulties, as sometimes siblings' needs often go unnoticed. Families also need to allow for their child's increasing independence, balanced with keeping their child within safe boundaries. More will be said in Chapter 7.

SEXUAL DEVELOPMENT

The cry of many parents is, 'What is normal?'. This is true for the area of sexual development. What the norm is today for mental health may not be the same as the norm from previous generations. Hopefully society has progressed from the days when a woman was considered 'mentally retarded' and locked away for having an illegitimate child. In the area of a child's sexual development, it is both curious and encouraging to note that parents have changed very little. They still believe in a child having a right to a childhood. At a recent conference in Winchester on sexual abuse it was made clear that paedophiles had a different construct, advocating the child's right to a sexual experience before the age of 8 years. Most of society would not agree with this.

Normal sexual play between non-abused children is mutually explorative and a way of finding out about body parts. It usually occurs between children of similar ages. Sexualised play from sexually abused children may not be the same sort of play. It may involve coercion or an older child, such as a teenager, abusing a younger child. Different levels of sexualised behaviour occur, such as digital penetration (fingers) to the vagina or anus, oral sex, simulated or actual sexual intercourse. Children who act out in this way may not actually have been sexually abused, although it is quite likely that they have learnt the behaviour from somewhere, possibly witnessing adult sexual intercourse in real life or on video.

The task of the occupational therapist who has been referred a child who has been sexually abused is, first, to accept the child and to work in partnership with non-abusing parents, to facilitate the child's emotional healing towards normal development. The occupational therapist may choose – with the child and carers – individual, family or group work approaches, depending on needs. The task is to build or restore a sense of trust, safety and boundary. There will be many emotions that the non-abusing carer may feel, such as guilt, loss of partner, low self-esteem, rejection of the child. The carer may need help in their own right from adult agencies or from child health agencies, if in connection with their parenting skills. The non-abusing father may need much help in managing sexualised behaviour from a daughter or son.

It has been suggested that, without intervention, children who have been abused will not integrate and understand their experience, and that boys in particular may go on to perpetrating

behaviour in a way that discharges their feelings of helplessness and impotency by allying with someone dominant. Occupational therapists are able to help children and adolescents by bridging the gap between the child's inner world and outer world by activity. Non-verbal communication is helpful to children and adolescents who find talking difficult, or who stammer as a result of their traumatic experiences or threats to keep silent.

This chapter does not have room to talk about child prostitution, other than to mention that it is worthy of further thought and discussion about how this affects the development of a child's mental health. More may be shared about treatment issues for children and adolescents who have been abused in Chapter 6.

MORAL AND SPIRITUAL DEVELOPMENT

Kohlberg (1987) was interested in how children arrived at the moral choices that they made. He formed a series of experiments for children of different ages and, whilst he was non-judgemental about the children's choices during the experiment, was curious to know the reasoning behind why the children made particular decisions. Kohlberg postured that there were three stages to child and adolescent development.

Stage 1: Preconventional morality (up to 8 years)

This, Kohlberg surmised, comprised two levels:

1. Punishment and obedience – the child desires to avoid being punished.

2. Instrumental relativism – the decisions the child makes are based on egocentric concerns or when, by obedience, the other person may give something that the child desires.

Stage 2: Conventional morality (9–10 years)

1. Social conformity – the child desires to fit in with society and therefore internalises some of society's values (e.g. no hitting at school).

2. Law and order – the child is concerned with how to interpret fairness and may be upset to discover that peers, siblings, parents, etc. have been cheating.

Stage 3: Post-conventional morality (11 years +)

1. Relativistic thinking – the child moves on from the issue of obedience to be more experimental in the thinking process. The child considers what is right and wrong for different situations.

2. Social contracts – the young adult has an awareness of the legal consequences of bad behaviour, and this awareness helps society's values to be internalised, providing a foundation for the person's own reasoning about moral decision-making.

Piaget's theories of the child's cognitive development, from concrete thinking to abstract reasoning, underpins Kohlberg's stages of moral development in children.

In his book *How to really know your child and help your child grow into spiritual maturity*, Ross Campbell, a child psychiatrist, considers spirituality as one part of the whole person, and very much influenced by the personality. He describes children in terms of being physical, emotional, psychological and spiritual beings. 'The way a child is helped to handle anger, frustration and his natural anti-authority behaviour during his teen years will affect him spiritually in exactly the same way that it affects him physically, emotionally and psychologically' (Campbell 1995, p. 18).

Campbell believes that children who develop an anti-parent/anti-learning attitude will be anti-spiritual. He advises that parents need to practise love and spirituality in order for the children to develop these principles. He postulates that unconditional love develops a wholeness within the child and helps the child to become self-confident. One of the ways to help children develop a good sense of self-esteem is for the parents to nurture this within themselves. He believes that parents who love themselves can give their children a good role model and that unconditional love is necessary for children to

develop to their maximum potential. He states in his book that he believes the best way to teach a child is by example, whether that is by the parents or main care-givers or by role models in education. His opinion is that rebellion in a child may come from the adults in the child's life giving the child the message: 'Do as I say, rather than as I do'. Campbell's conclusion is that parents who wish to instil spiritual values in their children need to live a spiritual life. He gives an example of a father who is fraudulent and then becomes angry when his child cheats on a school test, having learnt cheating behaviour from the father.

Of relevance to occupational therapists are Campbell's words to parents that they need continually to make their spiritual attitudes obvious to their children in their activities of daily living. Spirituality may develop in children whose parents have learnt about their idiosyncrasies and have taken the time to show them that they love them unconditionally. He refers to the stage of adolescent where youngsters are expressing their emotional hunger in the form of conformity with their peer group. In his book Campbell quotes that 54% of parents of 10-year-olds display little positive physical or verbal attention daily to their children, and that only 32% of parents of 14-year-olds give their children positive and physical attention. There is a great emphasis on the role that parents or the main care-giver has to play in bringing their children up to have spiritual values, and that much is based on the parents' practice of these values, particularly in relation to how they express their values through parenting.

Anger is seen as spiritual, and the way in which the child is reared with eye contact, focused attention and physical contact in a firm, love-based relationship can reduce a child's anger. Campbell believes that children must learn some guilt in order to develop a conscience, yet too much guilt can be damaging to them, and children need to know that they are forgiven. Parents telling their child to be quiet may cause the child's anger to be crammed deep inside an individual, and problems may emerge later on. Young children will express anger immaturely, but as they mature they need help to learn how to express anger in a more positive way.

There has been much recently in the news concerning the responsibilities of carers, education and the church in teaching children moral values and right from wrong. There are many schools of thought surrounding this, from relativistic thinking about what is right for you or the situation, to more fundamental values. There has been considerable debate in occupational therapy about the role of the occupational therapist in helping the individual to meet spiritual needs. For an individual to be self-actualised, it is helpful to have an understanding of Maslow's 'hierarchy of needs' in as much as the individual's physiological needs for food, water, rest, air and warmth, and needs for shelter and safety, combined with needs for love and belonging, self-esteem and significance, go before the need for self-actualisation, which is about individuals meeting their needs through actualising their personal goals. If the lower level needs are unfulfilled, the individual will not be ready to progress towards higher levels. In order to be fulfilled spiritually, the child's basic needs of a home, clothes and food, love and nurture need to be fulfilled.

Children seen in the occupational therapy department and child psychiatry come with a range of difficulties including antisocial behaviour such as stealing, bullying, and non-compliance at home and in the classroom. Knowledge of the stages of a child's moral development will help professionals to assess what level the child is functioning at, and in the formulation of a treatment plan; the occupational therapist advises on the next sequence of development relative to the child's chronological age and thinking process. The activity needs to be graded and not too difficult for the child.

REFERENCES

Atkinson R L, Atkinson R C, Smith E, Ben D, Nolen-Hoeksema S 1999 Hilgard's introduction to psychology, 13th edn. Harcourt Publishers, New York
Campbell R 1995 How to really know your child and help your child grow into spiritual maturity. Scripture Press.
Case-Smith J, Allen A S, Nurse-Pratt P (eds) 1996 Occupational therapy for children, 3rd edn. Mosby, St Louis
Kohlberg L 1987 Child psychology and childhood education. Longman, Harlow
Minuchin S 1977 Families and family therapy. Routledge, London

FURTHER READING

Butterworth G, Harris M 1994 Principles of developmental psychology. Psychology Press, Philadelphia

Davenport G C 1994 An introduction to child development, 2nd edn. Collins Educational, New York

Raynor E 1978 Human development. George Allen and Unwin, London

Spencer Pulaski M A Your baby's mind and how it grows. Cassell, London

Sylva K, Lunt I 1982 Child development – a first course. Blackwell, Oxford

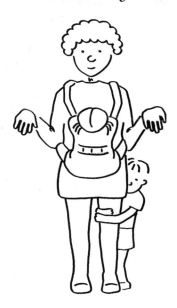

5

Attachment theory

Carol Hardy   Karin Prior

INTRODUCTION

Attachment theory has been developing for over 40 years now, and many occupational therapists will be familiar with some of its concepts, such as bonding, attachment and secure base, or the name of John Bowlby. In terms of guiding clinical practice, however, it seems that the potential of attachment theory has yet to be realised, not only for occupational therapy but for the specialty of child and adolescent mental health more generally.

Attachment theory offers a framework for understanding certain aspects of human relationships and the behavioural and emotional responses that accompany these. It considers the implications that attachment relationships have for a child's development, including their functioning, and provides a way of thinking about individual patterns of relating and the more problematic aspects of these.

This chapter provides an overview of attachment theory, beginning with a summary of the work of its cofounders, John Bowlby and Mary Ainsworth. Classification systems, systemic links and the recent research linking attachment with neurobiology are then discussed, followed by age-related concepts. Insecure patterns of attachment are explored along with a discussion of high-risk groups and clinical populations. Clinical applications of attachment theory follow, with the final section offering ideas on how to integrate concepts and research findings with an occupational therapist's work.

ORIGINS OF ATTACHMENT THEORY*

John Bowlby

From the beginnings of his career, John Bowlby was interested in the social–emotional environments in which children lived and the influence this had on their development. He considered actual events and, in particular, the ways in which children are treated to be more significant than other psychoanalytical theorists had at that time. His early papers, 'Forty-four juvenile thieves: their characters and home life' published in 1944 and the World Health Organization's report *Maternal Care and Mental Health* in 1951, linked maternal deprivation and deviant personality development, the latter including recommendations for the prevention of mental health adversity.

Bowlby valued scientific methods, and his early studies involved systematic observations of young children being separated from their parents, particularly when admitted to hospital or residential nursery. The impact of witnessing the children's distress first hand prompted researcher James Robertson, along with Bowlby, to create and publish the influential film 'A Two Year Old Goes to Hospital'. This led to wider recognition of the effects of early separations as well as reforms in hospital policy.

Bowlby began to formulate his theory in 'The nature of the child's tie to his mother', published in 1958. His ideas were influenced by ethology, and he drew comparisons between animal and human behaviour, noting that younger children tended to keep close to others who were stronger and more able to cope, like the young of many animal species, and to seek further proximity under situations of threat. He proposed that attachment behaviour and its complement, caregiving, are instinctive behaviours that serve a protective function, ensuring the survival of individuals and the species.

Bowlby conceptualised attachment as a behaviour control system, operating to maintain an acceptable distance or accessibility between the subject and their specific attachment figure. He saw attachment behaviours in the infant as developing through four phases along with corresponding changes in the care-giver's behaviour and becoming increasingly organised externally and internally. He proposed that 'internal working models' are gradually constructed from everyday interactions with attachment figures, influencing perceptions of self and others, and guiding behaviour. These may be conscious or unconscious, as is the case in early representations or those formed during painful moments and defensively

---

* For a more detailed overview see Bowlby (1988) and Bretherton (1991).

excluded from consciousness. Bowlby viewed internal working models as gaining increasing stability, such that new experiences and information, unless repetitive in nature, are likely to be altered to fit the individual's model rather than the model being reorganised to accommodate it.

Society's view of dependency and of the intense emotions that accompany attachment behaviour has been, and still continues at times to be, disapproving. Bowlby attempted to show that these are normal human responses that occur in children and adults. He argued, for example, that separation anxiety, anger and mourning are appropriate and functional responses to a threat of – or actual – separation and loss. Bowlby viewed the way in which others responded to a child's attachment behaviour as particularly influential in terms of whether a child is able to cope or develops pathological responses such as detachment, violence or unresolved grief (Bowlby 1980, 1991).

Mary Ainsworth

Mary Ainsworth's interest in individual differences amongst children's responses grew from her involvement in the early separation studies with Bowlby. She went on to do naturalist observations of infant–mother pairs in Uganda and Baltimore. She documented their interactions and attachment behaviours, and devised a classification system that recognised differences amongst infants as well as the mothers. Her results demonstrated a positive correlation between maternal sensitivity in the first year and infant attachment security (Bowlby 1991, Bretherton 1991).

To study the relationship between attachment and exploratory behaviour, Ainsworth designed an observation laboratory procedure called the 'Strange Situation' (see below). She found that infants explored the playroom and toys more when in the presence of their mother than they did when alone or with a stranger. Ainsworth later described this as a 'secure base' phenomenon, wherein the infant feels secure to move away knowing the care-giver is available and accessible if needed.

Using the Strange Situation in combination with home observations, Ainsworth defined further criteria for the classification of attachment behaviour. She found a correlation between reunion behaviour and the quality of the pair's

Table 5.1 The Strange Situation test	
Pattern of classification	**Infant's organisation of attachment behaviour towards primary care-giver**
Secure (B)	Uses parent as secure base to explore Shows signs of missing parent (e.g. searching, crying) when parent leaves Welcomes parent on return and seeks contact or interaction Easily comforted and soon returns to play
Insecure-avoidant (A)	Shows few or no obvious signs of distress when left Focuses on toys/environment, appearing competent but with neutral affect Avoids parent on return, especially after second absence May treat stranger in more friendly way than parent
Insecure-ambivalent (C) (also referred to as insecure-resistant)	Very distressed by separation Alternately seeks and resists proximity/contact with parent Difficult to comfort Some infants are markedly angry, others passive
Insecure-disorganised (D)	No clear behavioural strategy In presence of parent may show sequentially contradictory behaviour (e.g. distress at separation then expressionless backing away at reunion), simultaneous contradictory behaviours (e.g. clinging while sharply averting gaze), freezing/stilling, stereotypies/odd movements, undirected or misdirected movements/expressions (e.g. cries at stranger's leaving and attempts to follow), apprehension/fear, etc.
Compiled from Bowlby (1997) and Main & Solomon (1990).	

Table 5.2 The Adult Attachment interview

Classification	Characteristics of adult's narrative
Autonomous-secure	Coherent Internally consistent Links past to present
Dismissing-detached	Importance of attachment experiences is minimised Not much elaboration Limited memories Idealisation along with denial of negative experiences
Preoccupied-entangled (also referred to as enmeshed)	Preoccupation with attachment figure, past Lengthy, confusing stories Angry or passive content
Unresolved-disorganised (assigned in conjunction with one of above categories)	Lapses in monitoring of reasoning when discussing potentially traumatic events Lapses in monitoring discourse processes so that orientation to usual conversational structures is absent Reports of extremely disorganised/disoriented behavioural responses without any indication of later successful resolution

Compiled from Heard & Lake (1997), Holmes (1997) and Main & Hesse (1990).

relationship as observed at home, and showed that defensive processes could arise not only from prolonged separations but also from daily interactions.

CLASSIFICATION OF ATTACHMENT BEHAVIOUR

The 'Strange Situation' is a standardised assessment originally devised for 12-month-old infants (for a full description see Ainsworth et al 1978). It presents the infant with an unfamiliar setting and involves two brief separations from mother, first in the presence of a stranger and then alone. The infant's reactions to separation and reunion are then rated from a videotape and classified. The four major categories include: secure (B), insecure-avoidant (A), insecure-ambivalent (C) and insecure-disorganised (D) (Table 5.1).

The Adult Attachment Interview (AAI) developed by Mary Main and her colleagues is another well-known attachment classification procedure. It is a semistructured interview which requires participants to answer questions about their childhood experiences and relationships with their parents, so as to assess their internal working models of attachments. The coherence of the narrative is more important than the content in determining whether the participant is classified as autonomous-secure, dismissing-detached, preoccupied-entangled or unresolved-disorganised (Table 5.2).

Other procedures have been developed for age groups between infancy and adulthood. Some are behavioural, such as the 6-year Reunion Test (Main & Cassidy 1988), but many are representational. A family drawing task for children (Fury, Carlson & Sroufe 1997), an attachment story completion task for 3-year-olds (Bretherton, Ridgeway & Cassidy 1990) and the Inventory of Adolescent Attachment (Armsden & Greenberg 1987) are some examples.

THE ATTACHMENT BEHAVIOURAL SYSTEM AND ITS RELATIONSHIP TO OTHER SYSTEMS

The interrelationship between the attachment (care-seeking) system and other self systems has been extended by Dorothy Heard and Brian Lake (1997). Some of the systems function to regulate and maintain psychological and physical homeostasis, such as interpersonal care-seeking and care-giving or the defensive intrapersonal components of the care-seeking and sexual systems.

Others, such as exploration and interest-sharing with care-givers/peers, or the reproductive and affectionate components of the sexual system, are responsible for growth and development. Although the latter promote the development of competencies, thus furthering self-confidence and vitality, they depend on a level of homeostasis being maintained. Therefore, inadequate support or threat to an individual's physical or emotional well-being can interfere with creative exploration, maintaining companionable or sexual relationships, or providing nurturance, in that when stress is too great the care-seeking or defensive systems easily override these.

ATTACHMENT AND THE BRAIN

Research into brain development and functioning increasingly is providing scientific evidence to support some of the fundamental constructs of attachment theory. Neurobiological discoveries reveal that the physical structure of the brain is determined not only by genes that lay down the basic circuitry in the developing embryo, but by the neuronal activity that occurs after birth in the context of experiences (Begley 1997, Nash 1997). Connections or synapses are established through the electrical 'firing' of neurons in response to repeated sensory experiences, and those that are rarely used are eventually eliminated. Quality and frequency of experiences are therefore major determinants in the unique organisation of an individual's brain. Given that the brain's rate of growth is highest and its malleability greatest in the first few years of life, it is during these early years that the infant is at its most vulnerable with regard to the influence of experience. As Bruce Perry (1998, p. 2) has pointed out: 'The relative impact of time – time lost or time invested – is greatest early in life'.

Much early experience takes place in an interpersonal context with a care-giver. In sensitive and responsive care-giving, the adult acts as a regulator of the infant's state, providing opportunities for positive affect, minimising negative states such as distress or over/underarousal, and helping the infant to regain a more positive state after a negative intrapersonal or interpersonal experience.

These positive social experiences are considered to be critical to the development of the brain and to underlie the establishment of the attachment bond (Shore 1997). In contrast, prolonged experience of negative states, deprivation or repeated exposure to threat can interfere with normal brain development. For example, experiences of physical abuse early in life can result in abnormal stress responses, while emotional neglect can result in atypical patterns of neural activity that affect the areas of the brain responsible for empathy, humour, attachment and affect regulation (Perry et al 1995).

Neurobiological structuring of the brain is linked with the concept of 'internal working models', in that research from both bodies of knowledge suggests that experiences in the first year lay the foundation for later development and functioning. Allan Shore (1997) has described how early social experiences are stored as interactive representations in the orbital prefrontal areas of the brain and contain information pertaining to the parent and external environment, as well as to internal emotional and bodily states of the infant. He has identified the right cortical hemisphere as being more primitive and earlier to mature than the left, so that the earliest interactions are 'only registered in the deep unconscious' yet 'shape the individual's adaptive or maladaptive capacities to enter into all later emotional relationships'.

ATTACHMENT ISSUES AT DIFFERENT AGES
Birth to 6 months

One of the challenges of these early months is for the mother[†] and infant to develop ways of being together that are predominantly satisfying to them both, thereby ensuring that the infant's needs are met through the mother's ongoing desire to care for her infant. For the infant at this stage of life, basic physiological needs such as those for food and warmth must be attended to for survival, but regulation of internal states and sharing of affective experiences are also vitally

---

† The primary care-giver is referred to as mother to reflect the research studies and literature.

important for the development of homeostasis and the forming of an attachment bond.

The infant contributes to the attachment through instinctual and later learned behaviours which become increasingly organised and directed preferentially. For example, crying, smiling, clinging and babbling increase the likelihood of the infant keeping close to the mother. Infants, however, differ considerably in their capacities as a result of their genetic predisposition and their experiences prenatally and at birth, and thus in the contribution they make to the attachment relationship. An infant who is overly sensitive to sensory stimulation, for example, may require a different response from the mother than infants who are interested in their surroundings and easily establish means of self regulation. The Neonatal Behavioural Assessment Scale (Brazelton 1984) offers a qualitative measure of infant competency and can be used to help parents recognize the uniqueness of their newborn.

Mothers also differ in terms of what they bring to the relationship with their infant and the care they are able to provide. Past experiences or 'ghosts in the nursery' (Fraiberg, Adelson & Shapiro 1980) (i.e. having received inadequate parental care themselves or unresolved traumas), current stresses (i.e. a violent partner, recent loss or trauma), immaturity, lack of support, or physical or mental illness are some of the factors that can be influential in the parent–child relationship.

Although the interaction between the infant–mother pair is influenced by each member, it does seem that it is the mother's ability to respond sensitively to the individual needs of her infant rather than the constitution of the infant that is most powerful in determining the quality of the attachment that develops between them. Subsequently, the quality of care required by constitutionally vulnerable infants in order to establish a secure attachment may be quite different from that needed in those who are less so (Belsky and Rovine 1987).

6 months to 2 years

In the latter half of the first year the attachment bond grows stronger and attachment behaviour in the infant becomes more organised and obvious. If all goes well, the infant seeks proximity with the attachment figure, protests if separated from her, and shows a more pronounced fear response to strange people or objects and to simple clues of danger or threat (Bowlby 1991). The mother's sensitivity and responsiveness to the infant's increasing range of communications (i.e. behaviours, emotional expressions, vocalisations) (Grossman & Grossman 1991) and the quality and quantity of her physical and social contact (Lowinger, Dimitrovsky & Strauss 1995) have been shown to be particularly important.

With increasing mobility and capacity to read mother's cues from a distance, the infant is able to move away and potentially encounter more challenging and dangerous situations. Given the infant's relatively limited capacities (e.g. to tolerate frustration, assess safety) the mother's availability (i.e. as a secure base) is necessary for security, emotional regulation and protection from external threat. Simultaneously, internalisation of the mother's support, reliability and responsiveness continues, along with her encouragement of appropriate exploration and protectiveness. These internal representations are more affective than cognitive in nature at this stage (Holmes 1993) and enable the infant to become more self-regulating, self-protective and confident in exploration (Lieberman & Pawl 1990).

By this stage it is typical for infants to have more than one person to whom they are attached, although there is usually a hierarchy with regard to preference. This is most obvious at times when the infant's needs are strongest. In the second year, inanimate objects may temporarily serve as transitional security objects, when the infant is apart from an attachment figure (Bowlby 1997).

2–5 years

The attachment relationship becomes more of a 'goal-corrected partnership' and reciprocal in nature around the third or fourth birthday, although sometimes a little earlier (Bowlby 1997). The preschooler begins to picture others as having separate goals, and over these years develops the capacity for simple perspective-taking, comprehending others' motivations and plans. Sometimes the goals may be shared and achieved through joint participation, while at other times conflicts mean that either child or parent attempts to influence the other. This involves more sophisticated means of communication, often involving language and negotiation, as well as more skilled plans based on cues and experience (i.e. increasingly complex internal working models). The child, for example, may try to prevent a separation through pleading or making guilt-inducing comments, while the parent may reason or bargain.

With an increasing capacity for representation and to think in terms of time and space, the preschooler is more able to tolerate separation from an attachment figure and can be comforted by explanations, even from a stranger. Fears and phobias intensify, and concerns about safety develop, both for themselves and others. Parents need to be emotionally available and responsive at times of need, including when their child may be more 'babyish' than usual, due, for example, to feeling unwell or changes in the family such as a new baby. Other skills such as being able to provide guidance and instruction are required of parents at this stage (Fagot & Pears 1996).

More time is spent in the company of others, particularly other young children, and the quality of preschoolers' primary attachment relationships is considered to influence the way they interact with peers (Cicchetti et al 1990).

School years

During these years, there is a shift in terms of relating more with other adults, such as teachers or friends' parents, who may serve as attachment figures in addition to their parents. The way in which children perceive and respond to these adults is influenced by the expectations they have of adults' capacity to act as care-givers. Children's attention and participation in class, security and academic competence (Jacobsen & Hoffmann 1997), and their tendency to report more openly about feelings and on relationship-oriented coping strategies (Grossmann & Grossmann 1991), have been linked to the quality of their attachment representations.

Further cognitive development means that by the age of 6 years children have the capacity to monitor their own thinking, memory and action and to recognise the privacy of thought. This appears, from preliminary findings, to be related to security in the attachment relationship (Main 1991), and to be an important function in self-awareness and relating with others, both peers and adults. Peer relationships are increasingly significant in schoolchildren's lives, and there is evidence to suggest that the ability to manage conflict with peers and to develop satisfying friendships is influenced by the quality of attachment to parents (Grossmann & Grossman 1991).

Adolescence

The process of relinquishing the primary attachment to parents begins in adolescence and continues into adulthood. It can leave the adolescent feeling very alone, particularly if other attachment relationships have not been formed, and it is during this period of transition, between adolescence and adulthood, that loneliness is experienced most frequently and most painfully (Weiss 1991).

During these years, a parallel process also usually occurs, whereby relationships with peers become more important not only for sharing of interests but also in their potential for providing support, understanding and contributing to the adolescent's sense of security. Close friendships may be formed which may or may not include a sexual relationship, and these friends may serve as attachment figures.

The quality of attachment relationships to both parents and peers has been shown to be related to self-esteem and life satisfaction in adolescence. Also, a secure relationship with parents may be influential in terms of acting as a buffer against the potentially damaging effects of negative life experiences and stresses (Armsden & Greenberg 1987, Greenberg, Siegel & Leitch 1983).

Adulthood

Adult attachment relationships typically take the form of couple relationships, although other relationships such as those with siblings, close friends, a therapist, or a continuing link with one's parents, may also be characterised by the expression of attachment needs (Weiss 1991). Adults often have more than one attachment relationship in their life at any one time, and numerous attachment bonds may be formed and severed through one's adult years. When these are primarily secure, they can play a protective role in psychological health and parenting (Kotler & Omodei 1988).

When adults (or adolescents) become parents, they become the care-giver in the attachment relationship and their internal representations of being cared for have particular relevance to the infant's development. Narrative features in mother's descriptions of their unborn infants (Benoit, Parker & Zeanah 1997) and in their prenatal AAI classifications (Fonagy, Steele & Steele 1991), for example, have been found to be predictive of infant security over a year later.

INSECURE ATTACHMENTS

Internal working models have a remarkable continuity and longitudinal studies show that established configurations tend to operate outside conscious awareness and therefore become automatic (Benoit & Parker 1994). This is not a problem for those children or adults with secure representations of themselves and others as there is flexibility in their approach to achieving their goals in a variety of everyday contexts. However, the unconscious aspects become more problematic for individuals who have developed the insecure types of internal working models which influence not only behaviour and feelings but also other areas of everyday functioning (e.g. cognition, memory, attention). Reorganisation or reconstruction of such models is difficult and 'resist dramatic change' (Bowlby 1980).

Insecure-avoidant (A) and insecure-ambivalent (C) patterns both have an adaptive and organised nature. This helps the infant or older child to manage adversity, both internal (e.g. anxiety, anger) and external (e.g. unpredictable, rejecting care-giver) by having a strategy to follow.

It is useful to consider how adaptive but insecure patterns (A and C classifications) or actual maladaptive insecure attachment patterns (insecure-disorganised (D) classifications) are formed. Both the helpful and unhelpful aspects of these need to be borne in mind.

Regulation of emotions or affects has been linked with the formation of attachment bonds. Jude Cassidy (1994) found a correlation between patterns in A and C attachment classifications and two restricted styles of emotional regulation: systematic suppression and systematic heightening of emotion. A major biologically driven goal in the first year is the maintenance of a relationship with the attachment figure, and therefore these affect regulation styles can be understood as achieving this goal.

Insecure-avoidant (A) pattern

Infants and children classified in group A systematically suppress emotion, particularly when most distressed. They often display a neutral affect that includes muting of positive emotion too. Emotional control is understood as the child's effort to minimise their investment in a relationship in which they have experienced too much rejection, yet are reliant for protection and survival.

Parents of anxious-avoidant children tend to show the 'dismissing-detached' adult attachment classification (AAI), and features of this dovetail with the child's behaviour and expression of feelings. Adults deny negative emotion or negative past experience and there is an absence of negative affective expression when recalling distressing events, i.e. there is a disconnection between cognitive representation and normal emotion. These adults tend to ignore their infants' attachment needs; they show a limited range of affective expression and join with their infants only if the latter is calm and content. They withdraw contact when the infant shows negative emotion and requires regulation and/or comfort. Some adults may show over-intrusive behaviour which aims to focus the infant/child on activity and away from their attachment needs.

When seen in the Strange Situation test at 1 year these children make efforts to interest themselves in activity immediately on reunion despite physiological measures (e.g. cortisol levels) showing they are more distressed than the secure children. This pattern is seen to continue at 3 years. In a laboratory game, the young children not only display no negative emotion when aware they have lost the game but are actually more likely to smile.

So, what are the benefits to the child and parent of minimal emotional expression? For the child they minimise their emotional arousal level to avoid active engagement with the parent, thereby reducing the risk of experiencing further rejection and loss (i.e. necessary proximity to the parent). The child's lack of demand for emotional relatedness helps the parent maintain their defensive state of mind in which strong feelings of a negative or vulnerable nature are avoided.

Temperament theorists have suggested that group A children are intrinsically less fearful (behaviour inhibition). This is not borne out by measuring the heart rate and cortisol levels in this group, A category children having as high or higher heart rates on separation than secure group B children, and higher cortisol levels for longer periods of reunion despite their apparent lack of distress.

Insecure-ambivalent (C) pattern

The affect regulation styles of infants and children classified as group C correlate closely with the systematic 'heightening of emotion' pattern. Infants in the Strange Situation test show high affect expression on separation and on reunion. This appears to be a strategy of making perpetual strong bids for parental attention as the parent's availability may cease if the infant relaxes or is calmed. Parental features (more often classified as 'preoccupied/entangled' in the AAI) include the adult being especially focused on attachment relationships in their own past and present, with much anger and distress continuing unresolved despite all this attention. The infant flags up these emotions himself and the parent responds with some attention, although it has been observed that these adults find it harder to help

the child regulate their emotional state, that they soothe their babies less in first few months of life and that they also try to focus the infant when highly distressed on activity straight away. This failure to help the child manage highly aroused states does not promote self-regulation in the child and this results in continual reminders of the child's connection and attachment to them, which fits the parent's own state of mind in relation to attachment. The child then maintains a kind of contact with the parent but to the detriment of being able to attend to their environment in a positive and adventurous way. It is thought that these children may attend selectively to the more frightening aspects of the environment, so that, whilst this is in keeping with their perception of losing connection with their parent if they are calm and quiet, it creates a distorted view of the world around them.

Under stress, group C children have higher heart rates or cortisol levels than some, but not all, group B children. However, temperament may not be the major influence as two studies on 'irritable' babies found that 84% and 75% of such were not classified as group C (Crockenberg 1981).

Insecure-disorganised pattern

A further group of children were classified as insecure under this D categorisation after many researchers, studying widely varying populations, found that 10–15% of the subjects could not be easily placed in A, B or C categories. Before the D classification, most of these infants had been placed in the secure B category, although several characteristics of the infants and children or their circumstances conflicted with this. These young children were seen then in a variety of situations, at home, in more and less structured activities, and have been considered to be less secure than the A and C classified children. The dominant reason for this is that they appear to have no organised strategy for achieving a type of attachment relationship with a care-giver as the other insecure groups do.

Contradictory behaviours in these children feature highly: approach to the parent quickly followed by withdrawal, proximity sought but without positive affect or behavioural stilling, incomplete movements or indirect communications, face covering, rocking, wetting. Overall these infants are observed to be highly anxious and/or depressed. These young children do not compare similarly to one another, as do children in groups A and C.

Contextual factors often linked with the 'difficult-to-classify' infants are known abuse and/or neglect within the family environment. Apart from children who are actually experiencing abuse, another distinguishing characteristic is that one of the care-givers will be classified as 'unresolved' (U) on the AAI, indicating significant unresolved traumas in their own past. This is thought to manifest itself in frightening or frightened behaviour on the parent's part as a result of traumatic memories being triggered by a current event (e.g. aspects of an interaction with their infant or child).

It is interesting to note that the majority of infants and children are classified as group D in the presence of only one of their care-givers. This is of particular significance if the young child's behaviour appears quite bizarre or stereotyped and is suggestive of organic or neurological disorder, but is absent when they are with their other parent (Main & Solomon 1990).

Children classified as group D are considered to be in a paradoxical situation, which underlies their confusion and disorganisation. They are simultaneously drawn to the care-giver who is causing them distress and anxiety, and at the same time are experiencing the impulse to flee from them as the source of that alarm. Their behavioural strategy collapses and they flounder, trying to resolve the unresolvable (Main & Hesse 1990). The younger the child, the less means are available to them to try to cope; for instance, infants who are still immobile are more likely to resort to a 'freeze' response linked with dissociative mechanisms. The consequences for the rapidly developing brain are significant.

The majority of maltreated infants and children are classified in the D category but there is a sizeable proportion, around 15%, in the normal population low-risk samples where children are found to be disorganised/disoriented (Van

Ijzendoorn & Bakermans-Kranenburg 1996). This suggests there are many families who could present at clinic where there is a second-generation effect from one or more of the parents living with an unresolved traumatic past. The introduction of the U category for parents and the D classification for infants and children has made sense of hitherto unexplainable discrepancies. This discrepancy disappeared when U and D categories were included.

Insecure patterns in older children

For the insecurely attached older child, careful observations of the quality and pattern of interactions with care-givers is crucial. For example, with the normal expectation of increased independence, an avoidant pattern may be too easily overlooked. Main & Cassidy's (1988) 6-year Reunion Test focused on the patterns of behaviour during reunion and found a strong concordance with patterns of such in infancy, although the specific behaviours were different. In this 2-hour test, child rating at the insecure end of the scale includes: avoidance of the parent; apparent anxiety and expressions of inadequate feelings; rejection of the parent or a punitive approach to them; overly bright response with subtle disorganised behaviour; care-giving; at times subtle parental response to the parent from the child.

Briefly, the general reunion patterns follow that an 'insecure-avoidant' (A) 6-year-old will avoid contact with the parent in a non-emotional undemanding way; an 'anxious-resistant' (C) child shows ambivalence about proximity along with more affect expressions of sadness, anger and/or fear; and the insecure-controlling (formally category D in the Strange Situation) will either control the child–parent interaction by confronting and strongly rejecting the parent or by attempting to care for them, with bright expressions and comforting or guiding responses.

Along with the 6-year Reunion Test, researchers have studied children's narratives and pictures as a way to access the more subjective, even unconscious, aspects of the older child's internal working model. Kaplan and Main have described features of 5–7 year olds' family drawing that are linked to secure and insecure classifications. Fury, Carlson & Sroufe (1997) described this work and, more recently, extended it with their own adaptations to a coding system for 8–9 year olds. They included the absence of positive affect on drawings as a poor indicator, which Main and Kaplan had not owing to the younger children they had studied. Very few factors were individually discriminating to specific classifications apart from arms drawn downwards being highly correlated with the anxious-avoidant group and a rating of 'lack of individuation' linked only with the anxious-resistant group. Details of characteristics linked with all four classification groups can be found in their paper. Their conclusion was that early attachment history and current emotional functioning were significantly linked to negative drawing outcome, when IQ was controlled for.

Studies of insecurely attached middle-age children and adolescents show that the subjective tapping of stories and picture themes along with present everyday functioning add significantly to tests focusing on the primary attachment relationships.

HIGH-RISK GROUPS AND CLINICAL POPULATIONS

Bowlby (1991) proposed that the main cause of psychopathology characterised by chronic anxiety and mistrust is inappropriate or inadequate response to an individual's attachment behaviour during childhood. There is a high proportion of insecure classifications in clinical populations but it is also known that many factors influence whether children develop emotional or behavioural problems that require professional input. For instance, in a study of preschool children (Erickson, Sroufe & Egeland 1985) both securely and insecurely attached children who later developed behavioural problems at 4.5–5 years of age were much more likely to have lived with mothers who had separated from their adult partner during the period of 18 months to 4 years in the child's life. There were also distinct mother–child interaction patterns that accounted for some secure children having behavioural

difficulties whilst some insecure ones had no behavioural difficulties. These exceptions to the rule are well documented in this study. It can often be difficult clearly to link cause and effect factors. Mary Main's ideas (Main & Goldwyn 1984) are helpful and realistic in suggesting that there is a continuum of childhood dysfunction and a continuum of how available, rejecting or abusive parents may be towards their infants and children.

Despite these exceptions from which we can learn, there is a clear body of evidence that links insecure attachment classifications in both parents and children in the population receiving child and adolescent mental health services (CAMHS). One study (Van Ijzendoorn & Bakermans-Kranenburg 1996) showed that, compared with the norm of around 60% secure adults, only 14% of parents in a child clinical sample were found to be classifed as secure. Some 41% of these parents were found to be in the 'dismissing' category and 45% in the 'enmeshed'. If the 'unresolved' category is added, the number of adults classified as 'dismissing' is reduced, and then the U and E categories are found to be strongly overrepresented in both adolescent and adult clinical samples and for parents in child clinical samples. Van Ijzendoorn & Bakermans-Kranenburg (1996) also analysed data from 12 studies and found a predictive clinical link between Adult Attachment Insecurity and children being seen as clinically disturbed.

Five attachment-related risk factors have been proposed by Mary Main (1996) to link with the development of mental disorders in children and adults:

1. Failure to form a secure attachment from 6 months to 3 years.
2. Organised forms of insecure attachments.
3. Major separations or permanent loss of significant attachment figures.
4. Disorganised-disoriented (D) pattern of attachment in response to abuse.
5. D attachment pattern as a second-generation effect of parents' past trauma.

Although the D category in children and the U classification for adults are indicative of greater disturbance, clinical status is not exclusively related to these, as shown by many areas of poor functioning and/or clinical disorders linked to the other two insecure categories. It is unclear what kinds of disorder are more linked with specific classification type. One hypothesis suggests that internalising problems such as depression would be more commonly linked with the C and E categories and that externalising problems (e.g. conduct disorder) would link with DS and A groups. However, studies have not shown such a systematic relationship, one depressed clinical group of adults showing a higher proportion of the 'dismissing' (DS) category, although a specific link was found in one 16-year longitudinal study (Warren et al 1997), where 'insecure-resistant' classification in infancy was linked to anxiety disorders later tested for in adolescence. The 'anxious-avoidant' (A) attachment status in infancy did not predict later anxiety disorder.

Many studies (Goldberg, Gotowiec & Simmons 1995, Lyons-Ruth, Easterbrooks & Davidson Cibelli 1997) have found that 'insecure-avoidant' children, classified as group A in infancy, are most likely to have internalising problems rather than externalising problems, contrary to earlier studies. However, these earlier studies did not include the 'disorganised' (D) category. Later findings do make sense when the strategy of the avoidant child is considered (i.e. to 'hold in' negative affects, which is the main characteristic of the internalising stance).

Maternal depressive symptoms in the first 5 years have been strongly linked in several studies (Downey & Coyne 1990, Lyons-Ruth, Easterbrooks & Davidson Cibelli 1997) with externalising and internalising child symptoms and an increase in insecurity in the attachment relationships. A high level of maternal depression shows a strong correlation to externalising problems later, and mild cognitive deficits. However, it has been argued (Lyons-Ruth, Easterbrooks & Davidson Cibelli 1997) that it is unlikely that the mild mental deficit could account for the disorganisation of the attachment relationship or the behaviour problems at 7 years as attachment distributions were found to be similar to the norm in a sample where major biological deficits occurred in children with conditions such as Down syndrome and cystic fibrosis.

Children classified as 'disorganised' in infancy do feature highly in a great number of studies of clinical populations. By 6 years these children have often organised a pattern of relating to the parent that is classified as controlling-punitive or controlling-care-giving with either a hostile and/or helpless parent. Group D children are highly represented in samples of maltreated children. They express catastrophic fantasies in narratives and drawings, are thought to be more at risk for dissociative disorders, links already having been made with dissociative behaviour in primary and secondary school by Carlson (Main 1996). D categorisation in infancy has been followed up after 17 years and the adolescents showed marked indices of psychopathology. Another study has linked D status to formal reasoning difficulties in adolescents.

One further insecure group has been noted that alternate between A and C strategies, which are called 'unclassified'. This group features again in clinical populations of abusive or abused individuals (Main 1996).

CLINICAL APPLICATIONS
Diagnosis

Attachment classifications do not constitute diagnoses of attachment disorders. Two major types of attachment disorder have been designated in the International Classification of Disease (ICD) 10 (i.e. Reactive, Disinhibited) and the *Diagnostic and Statistical Manual of Mental Disorders* (DSM-IV), but, as Zeanah, Mammen & Lieberman (1993) point out, the criteria limit attachment disorders to extreme situations and do not adequately represent the presentations of disordered attachments. They propose five major types of attachment disorder diagnosable between 1 and 5 years of age:

1. Non-attached.
2. Indiscriminant (e.g. socially promiscuous or reckless/accident-prone/risk-taking).
3. Inhibited (e.g. excessive clinging or compulsive compliance).
4. Aggressive.
5. Role-reversed attachment disorder.

Validation of these diagnoses and their criteria is needed, however.

Interventions for primary attachment relationships

Articles describing interventions based on attachment theory are relatively few and tend to focus on infancy. A study by Lieberman, Weston & Pawl (1991) applied attachment theory and research measures to test the effectiveness of an intervention for anxiously attached 12 month olds and their mothers. The year-long intervention used infant psychotherapy and was found to be effective in enhancing maternal empathy and interaction with the child, as well as decreasing toddler avoidance, resistance and anger. The mothers' own representations of attachment, however, were not assessed so it is unclear to what extent the direct focus on changing maternal internal representations was influential in producing the results (Zeanah, Mammen & Lieberman 1993).

Another therapeutic intervention for mother–infant dyads, based on attachment theory and research, is Project STEEP (Steps Toward Effective, Enjoyable Parenting) described by Farrell Erickson, Korfmacher & Egeland (1992). The therapeutic relationship is used as an opportunity to influence parents' maladaptive internal working models and, ultimately, the parent–infant relationship. Some of the strategies used (e.g. encouraging the mother to link her infant's experience with her own early memories, the therapist speaking for the infant's experience) are aimed at increasing the parent's understanding of the infant's needs and feelings, and gaining insights into how past experiences influence present relationships. A study of its effectiveness had begun at the time of writing, and findings were encouraging although not conclusive.

Regulatory disorders often are accompanied by anxious attachment and separation anxiety and it has been suggested that interventions should address both constitutional and interactional aspects of the problem (DeGangi & Greenspan 1997). This study compared a child-centred intervention that emphasised infant psychotherapy in parent–child play interactions and a structured developmental parent guidance approach in the treatment of 14–30-month-old infants' irritability and inattention. The results showed the former to be more effective in that the parents learned to follow and encourage their child's initiation and attention, and the dyads improved in their communication.

Interventions with fostered and adopted children

Attachment is a core issue for these children who have suffered the trauma of separation(s) and frequently have a history of problematic attachments. In the first instance they require a stable environment with a care-giver who can provide consistent parenting and who can become emotionally involved. Therapeutic work may then focus on helping the child to confront beliefs about needing to be in control of others in order to feel safe and learning to trust that there are adults who can be in charge without hurting. Parents may need help in learning techniques that work with these children, as the usual 'good-enough' parenting strategies are often ineffective and parent–child work is an important ingredient in promoting the attachment between them (Randolph 1997).

INTEGRATING THEORY WITH OCCUPATIONAL THERAPY PRACTICE

In this section aspects of the attachment status of the child and how this manifests in their attachment relationship with parents or significant care-givers, and correspondingly how the child may relate to the occupational therapist in assessment or treatment, is considered. Evidence has already been given to remind us that within a CAMHS clinical population there will be a disproportionately high number of children, adolescents and parents who have an insecure attachment model that influences their approach to one another and to outside figures, and that has a secondary influence on some task-based functioning.

Although there will be a greater or lesser influence from the attachment basis depending on the levels of adversity experienced in the past and currently, it is important to think about how the child and the parents may experience assessment or treatment interventions, and to consider what influence their attachment histories has on this. Noting the attachment behaviours, thought constructs, affect regulation and interactions will help to comprehend the child and/or family functioning. Thought is required on how our interventions may affect the relationship between the child and care-giver. In general, we need to be alert as to whether our interventions are having a positive influence on dysfunctional patterns or being negatively reinforcing.

Talking with parents

In CAMHS the high proportion of parents classified with an insecure attachment status will in turn correlate with the strong likelihood of these children having been already insecurely attached at 12 months of age. Some general points about talking with parents and seeing families together will be raised. Information is probably best gathered through direct contact where contextual information is available. If other professionals are to assess the family together, either observing this or questioning the colleague involved on attachment related issues will help to build a rounded view of the child's past and current experience of care and security.

It may not be possible to see first hand the patterns of interactions that influence the formation of a view of themselves, others and their environments. Therefore, when this is not available because of the older age of the child, an open mind is needed to question what previous contributing factors may have brought the child to need a professional service. The question arises as to what cannot be managed within the family context and for how long this has been the case. However, it can be possible through careful and gradual questioning to ask the parent, for exam-

ple, about how easily they considered they could influence the child when younger, at what age did this begin to be hard, how active the child was before this point in time when change was identified. The beginnings of self-asserted autonomy in an infant can be distressing for some parents who view this as a rejection, but for other parents it may be experienced as too demanding and controlling.

Much has been noted of the early interaction patterns that precede the onset of later symptomatic behaviour (for a review see Lyons-Ruth 1996). Some of this requires direct observation; for example, intrusive over-controlling parental behaviour towards the toddler is highly unlikely to be self-reported in hindsight by a parent who is angry and distressed by the difficult behaviour of their 6 year old. The meanings that the parent attributes to the early problems in relation to their child are revealing and help the understanding of what may have preceded the distressing negative cycle. This can be a complex and lengthy issue to deal with but may shed light on the child's current behaviour and provide opportunities for problems to be reframed and then approached differently by parents.

A number of characteristics have emerged from the many AAI studies (Main 1996, Van Ijzendoorn & Bakermans-Kranenburg 1996) that indicate a striking difference in the adults' quality of speech when discussing attachment-related topics compared with non-attachment topics. This may help to explain the discrepancy between the well organised, fluent account with which parents may present certain subjects (even including research on their child's symptomatology) and the difficulty in talking about significant relationships or experiences in their own past. Autobiographical memory may be fine as long as it is not related to attachment information, adults classified as in group DS even showing somewhat better memory capacity if non-attachment related. The significance of this for engaging the parents directly in work or to support individual child work is in their restricted capacity to tolerate dependency needs for themselves or their child.

Another area where the parent's report should be carefully noted is in their descriptions of the child's behaviour and/or emotional states. A study (Lyons-Ruth, Easterbrooks & Davidson Cibelli 1997) comparing teacher and parent reports (using the Child Behaviour Checklist, CBCL) found that teachers reported high CBCL externalising symptom scores for children whose mothers had a history of abuse or of being hospitalised, whereas the mothers of these children did not report such behaviours. It was also found that mothers of insecurely attached children significantly underreported their child's fearfulness and insecurity, a characteristic the author has repeatedly noted in the clinic when children seen as highly anxious by the clinician are nearly always reported as having no fear or worries by parents.

Working with children

As many different types of assessment and treatment intervention may be planned by the occupational therapist, one type of assessment will be illustrated for the purpose of mapping attachment concepts on to a process of therapeutic contact.

An informal play or activity session for a 7 year old will be used as an example, in which the occupational therapist is an unfamiliar adult. The occupational therapist may have specific areas of functioning to be assessed in depth which include the child's organisational skills, approach to activities, capacity for emotional regulation, responsivity to play and to the occupational therapist.

From an attachment standpoint, one of the first considerations would be whether or not to assess the child with or without the care-giver present, or alternatively to gain a comparison of the child's functioning in both circumstances if there are indicators to suggest this would be helpful. For example, this latter approach would be useful with a family in which a parent was anxiously overinvolved, the child appeared anxious/resistant and presented as inept with poor attention during play, whilst in their parent's presence. When seen individually a child can show a significantly higher level of cognitive/motor functioning and social communication.

The context(s) in which to assess the child may be decided by how available, practically and emotionally, each parent is. It is important to keep in mind that children's attachment to one parent may be secure whilst insecure to the other. Adult reporting of their partners or ex-partner's relationship to the child is not always reliable, either through a wish to protect the other or, conversely, a wish – sometimes unconscious – for the other to appear a less capable parent figure.

If there has not been a previous opportunity to see the child and parent(s) together, the occupational therapist will need to make a decision on how to proceed in the first instance but can use what would be the initial contact with parent(s) and child together to observe interaction and to discuss briefly with the parent how the child is feeling about the appointment. This is not to exclude the child but can reveal important information about the parent's understanding of the child's position (i.e. the parent's view or reaction to their child who is likely to be in a stressed state). A number of opinions and accounts may be heard from parents, for example whether and how the parent has prepared the child for the session, for a possible separation with themselves, to meet and spend time with an unfamiliar adult. How the parent expects the child to make the transition if there is to be a separation provides useful information (e.g. 'He doesn't care', 'He'll go with anybody', 'She didn't want to come and we haven't talked about it'). Parents, if in touch with their child's views, may remark on these and so an absence of any child perspective from the parent should be noted and can be explored further at a later date. Older children may or may not refer to their parents to check out things or for reassurance. The manner in which they separate from one another is often characteristic of the dyad's pattern of the relatedness; for example, an 'avoidant' child may without any reference, verbal or non-verbal, make a superficial but over-familiar connection with a worker and move away from their parent almost eagerly, whereas a group D child by 6 years will have somewhat organised their previously fragmented or contradictory behaviours and moved into the punitive or care-giving stance. Such children may attempt to reassure the parent that everything will be all right or try to guide the parent in a regulating manner, thereby reversing the usual child–parent roles. Withdrawn behaviour, for instance, may have different meanings according to the type of insecurity the child experiences, for example in 'insecure-avoidant' it can indicate a disconnectedness, whilst in 'insecure-resistant' it can link with passivity and more obvious fearfulness. Building up a picture during many scenarios is therefore crucial.

How children function and interact during the assessment itself will be influenced in part by their internal representations of themselves, which includes 'perceived competence'. Harter (1982) used this term to describe the combination of an individual's self-cognition (i.e. beliefs about the self that are descriptive and thought to be factual by the individual) and self-esteem, a more global judgement of the value of oneself. A securely attached child would have an expectation that in challenging situations (e.g. being assessed by an unfamiliar adult) help would be forthcoming should difficulties arise, as they are worthy of help. How a child expresses their ideas or feelings, carries things through into practice, and turns for and accepts help with a task will be dynamic factors pertinent in an assessment setting.

Outlines of prominent features that could appear within an assessment context, within the three major insecure classification groups, are described below.

Group A child

The child may fluctuate between appearing keen for attention, apparently wishing to make contact, and becoming distant, almost dismissive, of the adult's presence. Reciprocal communication may be short lived where the child perhaps initiates a conversation but soon responds with minimal replies. The child's affect may be neutral, even rather blank, but there are either flashes of anger or a sense of underlying strong anger. The child may persist for a short while with a difficulty, then give up and turn away without asking for any assistance, or they may make a bid for help and even appear overly dependent for a moment, before ignoring or dismissing the help

offered. Attention may be poor, the child leaving activities half finished but with little or no communication as to their thoughts behind it. There may be brief statements indicating that their actions are no good.

Group C child

The child may show heightened distress, anxiety or anger, especially if separation from the parent has occurred. They may appear overly preoccupied with the interpersonal contact and actions of the worker and so find it difficult to begin to focus on any activity. 'Giving up' may occur; a sense of helplessness and passivity around the activity and help offered may well receive responses that 'nothing can help' or that involve passing the activity over to the occupational therapist. Children may remain preoccupied with thinking about their parents and want to talk about this more than use the play materials available. This can mean that sessions need to be graded in time, according to the stage of assessment. Children may be very responsive to general background noise and show poor habituation to this.

Group D child

The child having separated from the parent with relative ease may then try to take control of the session and the worker's actions and behaviour too. This may occur by overt or covert actions on the child's part. Overtly the child may assume the position of authority, acting precociously in either a caring or a critical way. More subtle control is experienced when a child appears cut off, watchful and relatively unresponsive. Approach to activities may have a particularly rapid start–stop quality and, if interest from the occupational therapist is shown towards the child's actions, this appears to have an off-putting effect as the child ceases that activity. In general there may be a poverty of imaginative or affective quality to any play or activity; for example, play figures may be acting out dangerous or frightening scenarios in an automatic manner with no affect expressed or acknowledged for them. Whilst playing, the child may display a blank facial affect themselves. If the child does communicate verbally, the discourse may have frequent pauses or interruptions (i.e. 'false starts') or may be delivered in such a way that does not expect a response or encourage two-way communication. If the worker does respond, the child may ignore it and start a new topic.

CONCLUSION

Attachment theory has a lot to offer clinicians from its grass-roots ideas and concepts to the expanding scientific research and study across the age span. Its relevance to every individual in terms of instinctive attachment behaviour and the development of internal working models has been shown. Although insecure attachment status does not necessarily link directly with a clinical disorder, many examples have highlighted the relevance of this status for the clinical population seen in everyday work. The authors hope that it will interest occupational therapists to explore further the ongoing research findings that are providing answers to some of the complex presentations of difficulties seen in the CAMHS field.

REFERENCES

Ainsworth M D S, Blehar M C, Waters E, Wall S 1978 Patterns of attachment: a psychological study of the strange situation. Erlbaum, Hillsdale, NJ

Armsden G C, Greenberg M T 1987 The inventory of parent and peer attachment: individual differences and their relationship to psychological well-being in adolescence. Journal of Youth and Adolescence 16(5):427–451

Begley S 1997 How to build a baby's brain. Newsweek Spring/Summer:28–32

Belsky J, Rovine M 1987 Temperament and attachment security in the strange situation: an empirical rapprochement. Child Development 58:787–795

Benoit D, Parker K C H 1994 Stability and transmission across three generations. Child Development 65:1444–1456

Benoit D, Parker K C H, Zeanah C H 1997 Mother's representations of their infants assessed prenatally: stability and association with infant's attachment classifications. Journal of Child Psychology and Psychiatry 38(3):307–313

Bowlby J 1980 Attachment and loss, vol. 3: loss: sadness and depression. Hogarth, London

Bowlby J 1988 A secure base: clinical applications of attachment theory. Routledge, London

Bowlby J 1991 Attachment and loss, vol. 2: separation: anxiety and anger, 2nd edn. Hogarth, London

Bowlby J 1997 Attachment and loss, vol 1: attachment, 2nd edn. Pimlico, London

Brazelton T B 1984 Neonatal behavioural assessment scale, 2nd edn. Lippincott, Philadelphia

Bretherton I 1991 The roots and growing points of attachment theory. In: Murray Parkes C, Stevenson-Hinde J, Marris P (eds) Attachment across the life cycle. Routledge, London, p 9

Bretherton I, Ridgeway D, Cassidy J 1990 Assessing internal models of the attachment relationship. An attachment story completion task for 3-year-olds. In: Greenberg M T, Cicchetti D, Cummings E M (eds) Attachment in the preschool years. University Press, London, ch 9, p 273

Cassidy J 1994 Emotion regulation: influences of attachment relationships. Monographs of the Society for Research in Child Development 59(2–3):228–249

Cicchetti D, Cummings E M, Greenberg M T, Marvin R S 1990 An organisational perspective on attachment beyond infancy – implications for theory, measurement and research. In: Greenberg M T, Cicchetti D, Cummings E M (eds) Attachment in the preschool years. University Press, London, p 3

Crockenberg S B 1981 Infant irritability, mother responsiveness, and social support influences on the security of infant–mother attachment. Child Development 52(3):857–865

DeGangi G A, Greenspan S I 1997 The effectiveness of short-term interventions in treatment of inattention and irritability in toddlers. Journal of Developmental and Learning Disorders 1(2):276–298

Downey G, Coyne J C 1990 Children of depressed parents: an integrative review. Psychological Bulletin 108:50–76

Erickson M F, Sroufe L A, Egeland B 1985 The relationship between quality of attachment and behavior problems in preschool in a high-risk sample. Monographs of the Society for Research in Child Development 50(1–2):147–166

Fagot B I, Pears K C 1996 Changes in attachment during the third year: consequences and predictions. Development and Psychopathology 8:325–344

Farrell Erickson M, Korfmacher J, Egeland B R 1992 Attachments past and present: implications for therapeutic intervention with mother–infant dyads. Development and Psychopathology 4:495–507

Fonagy P, Steele H, Steele M 1991 Maternal representations of attachment during pregnancy predict the organization of infant–mother attachment at one year of age. Child Development 62:891–905

Fraiberg S, Adelson E, Shapiro V 1980 Ghosts in the nursery: a psychoanalytic approach to the problems of impaired infant–mother relationships. In: Fraiberg S (ed) Clinical studies in infant mental health. Basic Books, New York, p 164

Fury G, Carlson E A, Sroufe L A 1997 Children's representations of attachment relationships in family drawings. Child Development 68(6):1154–1164

Goldberg S, Gotowiec A, Simmons R 1995 Infant–mother attachment and behavior problems in healthy and chronically ill pre-schoolers. Development and Psychopathology 7:267–282

Greenberg M T, Siegel J M, Leitch C J 1983 The nature and importance of attachment relationships to parents and peers during adolescence. Journal of Youth and Adolescence 12(5):373–386

Grossmann K E, Grossman K 1991 Attachment quality as an organizer of emotional and behavioral responses in a longitudinal perspective. In: Murray-Parkes C, Stevenson-Hinde J, Marris P (eds) Attachment across the life cycle. Routledge, London, p 93

Harter S 1982 The perceived competence scale for children. Child Development 53:87–97

Heard D, Lake B 1997 The challenge of attachment for caregiving. Routledge, London

Holmes J 1993 John Bowlby and attachment theory. Routledge, London

Holmes J 1997 Attachment, autonomy, intimacy: some clinical implications of attachment theory. British Journal of Medical Psychology 70:231–248

Jacobsen T, Hofmann V 1997 Children's attachment representations: longitudinal relations to school behavior and academic competency in middle childhood and adolescence. Developmental Psychology 33(4):703–710

Kotler T, Omodei M 1988 Attachment and emotional health: a life span approach. Human Relations 41(8):619–640

Lieberman A F, Pawl J H 1990 Disorders of attachment and secure base behaviour in the second year of life. In: Greenberg M, Cicchetti D, Cummings M (eds) Attachment in the preschool years. University Press, London, p 375

Lieberman A F, Weston D R, Pawl J H 1991 Preventative intervention and outcome with anxiously attached dyads. Child Development 62: 199–209

Lowinger S, Dimitrovsky L, Strauss C 1995 Maternal social and physical contact: links to early infant attachment behaviors. Journal of Genetic Psychology 156(4):461–476

Lyons-Ruth K 1996 Attachment relationships among children with aggressive problems: the role of disorganised early attachment patterns. Journal of Consulting and Clinical Psychology 64:64–73

Lyons-Ruth K, Easterbrooks M A, Davidson Cibelli C 1997 Infant attachment strategies, infant mental lag, and maternal depressive symptoms: predictors of internalizing and externalizing problems at age 7. Developmental Psychology 33(4): 681–692

Main M 1991 Metacognitive knowledge, metacognitive monitoring, and singular (coherent) vs. multiple (incoherent) model of attachment: findings and directions for future research. In: Murray-Parkes C, Stevenson-Hinde J, Marris P (eds) Attachment across the life cycle. Routledge, London, p 127

Main M 1996 Introduction to special section on attachment and psychopathology: 2. Overview of the field of attachment. Journal of Consulting and Clinical Psychology 64(2):237–243

Main M, Cassidy J 1988 Categories of response to reunion with parent at age 6: predictable from infant attachment classifications and stable over a 1-month period. Developmental Psychology 24(3):415–426

Main M, Goldwyn R 1984 Predicting rejection of her infant from mother's representation of her own experience: implications for the abused–abusing intergenerational cycle. Child Abuse and Neglect 8(2):203–217

Main H, Hesse E 1990 Parents' unresolved traumatic experiences are related to infant disorganized attachment status: is frightened and/or frightening parental behavior the linking mechanism? In: Greenberg M T, Cicchetti D,

Cummings E M (eds) Attachment in the preschool years. University Press, London, p 161

Main M, Solomon J 1990 Procedures for identifying infants as disorganised/disoriented during the Ainsworth strange situation. In: Greenberg M T, Cicchetti D, Cummings E M (eds) Attachment in the preschool years. University Press, London, p 121

Nash J M 1997 Fertile minds. Time February 10:51–58

Perry B D 1998 Biological relativity: time and the developing child. Baylor College of Medicine, Houston, Texas

Perry B D, Pollard R A, Blakeley T L, Baker W L, Vigilante D 1995 Childhood trauma, the neurobiology of adaptation, and 'user-dependent' development of the brain: how 'states' become 'traits'. Infant Mental Health Journal 16(4):271–291

Randolph E 1997 Children who shock and surprise: a guide to attachment disorders, 2nd edn. RFR Publications, Kittredge, Colorado

Shore A N 1997 Interdisciplinary developmental research as a source of clinical models. In: Moskowitz M, Monk C, Kaye C, Ellman S (eds) The neurobiological and developmental basis for psychotherapeutic intervention. Jason Arsonson, Northvale, New Jersey, p 2

Van Ijzendoorn M H, Bakermans-Kranenburg M J 1996 Attachment representations in mothers, fathers, adolescents, and clinical groups: a meta-analytic search for normative data. Journal of Consulting and Clinical Psychology 64(1):8–21

Warren S L, Huston L, Egeland B, Sroufe A 1997 Child and adolescent anxiety disorders and early attachment. Journal of American Academy of Child and Adolescent Psychiatry 36(5):637–644

Weiss R S (1991) The attachment bond in childhood and adulthood. In: Murray Parkes C, Stevenson-Hinde J, Marris P (eds) Attachment across the life cycle. Routledge, London, p 66

Zeanah C H, Mammen O K, Lieberman A F 1993 Disorders of attachment. In: Zeanah C H (ed) Handbook of infant mental health. Guilford, New York, p 332

FURTHER READING

Cassidy J, Berlin L J 1994 The insecure/ambivalent pattern of attachment: theory and research. Child Development 65:971–991

George C 1996 A representational perspective of child abuse and prevention: internal working models of attachment and caregiving. Child Abuse and Neglect 20(5):411–424

Isabella R A 1993 Origins of attachment: maternal interactive behavior across the first year. Child Development 64:605–621

Main M, Kaplan N, Cassidy J 1985 Security in infancy, childhood and adulthood: a move to the level of representation. Monographs of the Society for Research in Child Development 50(1–2):66–104

RESOURCES

International Attachment Network
6 Oman Avenue
London
NW2 6BG

- courses, workshops
- news bulletin.

Adoption UK
(formerly Parent to Parent Information on Adoption Services, PPIAS)

Lower Boddington
Daventry
Northamptonshire
NN11 6YB
Tel: 01327 260 295

- information, support and advice to prospective and existing adoptive parents and long-term carers
- information for professionals on attachment issues and adoption (resource packs, booklets, booklists, etc.).

6

The therapeutic use of play

Pauline Blunden

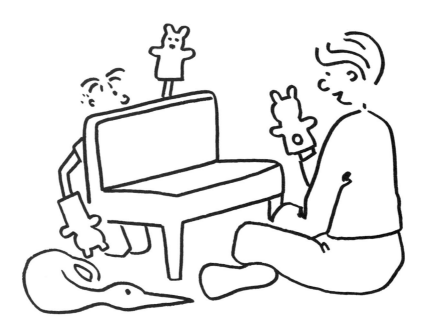

CHAPTER CONTENTS

INTRODUCTION

This chapter is intended to give a brief overview of the therapeutic use of play. Within the space available it cannot be exhaustive and other play therapists may choose different approaches to study the subject.

Many different disciplines practise play therapy; in this chapter I have tried to link the practice with occupational therapy. Practical aspects of running play therapy sessions are discussed, as well as some of the most commonly referred psychiatric disorders. The theoretical background to play therapy is touched upon here and in other chapters in this book.

beneficial to have joint play therapy sessions with the carers and child together if it is found in the play therapy assessment that the child can concentrate well during the sessions and at school, but remains restless in the home situation.

It is important to find out when the behaviours began. Many changes in a child's life can precipitate these behaviours, for example changes of school, bereavement, moving house, changes in home situation. The reasons may not be known, but if the behaviours began at a certain time, it is useful to explore with the carers what may be the precipitating factor.

Focused play therapy can then be used to address the child's trauma and, at the end of therapy, to assess whether the child's concentration has improved and distractibility lessened. Further activity sessions may be necessary to improve the length of the child's concentration span but, when the underlying reason is addressed, this is often not necessary.

Children abused physically, sexually or emotionally

Children who have been abused are usually seen for play therapy after the abuse has been disclosed and investigated, and when they are no longer in contact with the abuser and are in a safe situation at home. Sometimes the abuse may have happened several years before it is disclosed and the child may present with flashbacks to the abuse, emotional and behavioural disturbances, psychosomatic and interpersonal difficulties.

Children who have been sexually abused may have blurred role boundaries, be promiscuous, have a lack of trust, and feel themselves permanently damaged and different from their peers. All abused children have low self-esteem and many are very angry, but may not know how to display the anger safely.

Play therapy for these children may be long term and is often non-directional in nature, encouraging the expression of genuine feelings and allowing the child to build a relationship with an adult where the child has the power to choose and make decisions and the adult can be trusted. The OT will be aiming to give the child back a sense of self by empowering the child and allowing the child true expression of their feelings. The child will learn skills in coping with stress and, in the case of a sexually abused child at the end of therapy, specific work is undertaken to teach the child to know what are safe boundaries.

Children may need further therapy at a different developmental age. Play therapy can address the child's distress only at their present level of functioning; for example, a child who has play therapy to address the trauma of sexual abuse at the age of 5 years may need further specialised counselling or group work when a teenager to address the issues arising at that age.

Stressful life events that are unresolved

Children referred with loss issues arising from unresolved life events, such as bereavement, fostering, trauma and parental separation, may well have experienced faulty attachment and unsatisfactory parenting. Parallel work by another clinician may need to be done with the carers whilst the child is having play therapy. The child may present as low in mood, often tearful, a loner, unable to express grief, fear or anger, sometimes overactive and with inability to concentrate, usually with low self-esteem. Some children present with eating difficulties, i.e. under- or overeating to compensate for their loss. There may also be somatic symptoms such as stomach aches.

Play therapy needs to be individually tailored to each child. It is well known that depression in adulthood often goes back to unresolved grief in childhood. Some children present with many stressful life events and, by taking a non-directive approach, the child is able to work on the events and situations that are most troubling at the time of the referral.

Small group work is possible where there are several children suffering from the same loss issues (e.g. abnormal bereavement reactions); a parallel group is often run for the parents of these children, who may need group counselling themselves. Some children may not feel strong enough emotionally to join a group, and are then given individual play therapy and moved into group work later.

Children experiencing post-traumatic stress

These children are often referred as part of the process of debriefing from a traumatic incident. Specialist post-trauma debriefing may have been done with other family members, but the child may be too young or too traumatised to cope with verbal debriefing and may need to use the language of play to express feelings about the incident.

Sometimes these children have bad dreams about the traumatic incident or may have generalised their fear into other objects; for example, a child who was nearly trapped in a car on fire may not be able to go in lifts or into an enclosed space with the door shut, but has no trouble travelling in cars. Children like this may say they cannot remember the incident or they may avoid anything that reminds them about what happened. The child may regress and begin wetting and soiling or become uninterested or preoccupied. Sleep patterns are often changed and the child may be extra-vigilant and startled by loud sounds and sudden movements.

Focused play therapy, which is specifically chosen to help the child remember all of the trauma, and then gradual debriefing over a specific number of sessions is the treatment of choice. The child may have concentration and memory problems and be worried about repetitive thoughts about the trauma, which can occur at any time but are more often triggered off by environmental stimuli.

Focused play therapy is used with these children, who may be avoidant of the most disturbing parts of the trauma. Once the whole of the trauma has been explored using play therapy techniques, the child is often able to verbalise more of what they felt when the trauma happened and gain mastery over these feelings. In addition these children may need specific treatment for fears and phobias which may take the form of a desensitisation programme.

Poor peer relationships

Children presenting with any of the previously mentioned psychiatric disorders may have poor peer relationships. However, some children have this as a primary referral.

The OT assesses the child's cognitive, motor and visual perceptual skills, since, if these are poor, peer relationships are often also poor. When social skills are maladaptive, the child will often ask for reassurance from adults, show regressed behaviours and withdraw from situations in which compromise or cooperation with peers is necessary. Frequently these children are anxious and may try to avoid going to school.

Children with these problems are best helped in small groups which combine social skills with drama and shared activities.

PLAY THERAPY REFERRAL

In most cases the child will already have been assessed by the multidisciplinary team and a specific referral will have come to the therapist from the team. The OT may well decide to make her own assessment before deciding on her goals for play therapy. The initial assessment may take more than one session, depending on the severity of the difficulties and the extent of the information the therapist has already been given.

Before meeting the family and the child, the therapist may send out some information on play therapy to the carers so that they are able to prepare any questions they may wish to ask. Information sent to the carers would include:

- the name of the OT who will be seeing them and the place where the interview will take place
- any other information they may need to know about transport and parking
- an introduction to play therapy
- issues of confidentiality.

An *example of information sent to carers* is shown in Box 6.1.

Where does play therapy take place?

Ideally play therapy does not take place at home or school, but in a neutral room which is quiet and free from interruptions, with good lighting and no distracting view. The playroom must be safe, with clear physical boundaries. There should be an area where messy regressive play is possible (Fig. 6.4) and some kind of structure that has multiple uses as a puppet theatre, Wendy house (Fig. 6.5), police station, spaceship or whatever else the child wishes to use it for, to allow the child to find a secluded place and choose his or her own access. A waterproof floor, which can be easily swept around the messy play area, is needed, and a carpeted area should be available for sitting or lying in comfort. Tables and chairs need to be child height, as does the sink and shelves housing the sand-tray toys (Fig. 6.6). The room should feel welcoming, but not cluttered and overwhelming so that each section of the room creates a different type of space for the child to play in. A large walk-in cupboard is ideal to store the majority of the toys and provides a lockable place to put the children's artwork for safe keeping from one session to the next or to store a particularly significant con-

---

Box 6.1 Information for carers

INTRODUCTION

Play therapy sessions at the clinic are run by the occupational therapist (OT). These sessions may be on a one-to-one basis with a child, in a group situation with another member of staff, or with the carers present.

Adults can often explain how they feel, but many children do not find this easy. Children use play to understand their world and what is happening around them. Play therapy is a way of helping children use their own language of play to communicate their problems. Children who are having difficulties sometimes find it hard to understand or talk about a problem.

If your child is referred for play therapy, the therapist will explain the method of working, length of sessions, and timing of the next appointment, at the initial play therapy session.

GUIDELINES FOR CARERS

If your child is referred for play therapy on a one-to-one basis, it is important that the child is able to understand that therapy time is meant for them. The therapist is there to recognise the feelings the child is expressing and help them to gain insight into their problem.

If a child wants to tell an adult about what happened during a play therapy session, please listen to them. However, it is best not to question them or try to find out what happened in a session, since it is

important that the child feels that whatever is revealed during play therapy may remain private, where appropriate, amongst the clinic's multidisciplinary team.

Sometimes children may take unresolved issues away with them after the sessions, which will affect their behaviour; for example, they become withdrawn or overactive for a while. If this does happen, it would be helpful if the carers could notify the occupational therapist and, where possible, contain rather than discipline this behaviour.

It is important that a child should not be overloaded or confused by too many differing treatments or therapies. If a child is involved in play therapy it is advisable that no other in-depth work is carried out with that child unless specific agreement has been reached with all parties concerned.

CONFIDENTIALITY

Carers may feel concerned or left out when their child/children are involved in play therapy. Any carer who feels a need to talk about what is happening is welcome to ask for an appointment with the OT or other member of the clinic staff to discuss this, or maybe given parallel appointments with another member of the clinic staff whilst the play therapy is taking place.

. . . .

(signed) – Occupational Therapist

---

struction, for instance of Lego, which the child will use and add to at subsequent therapy sessions (Fig. 6.7).

Windows will need to have safety glass and catches and, if overlooked, blinds, which the child can pull down. Easy access to a toilet is important for most children.

The equipment and toys needed to furnish the playroom will depend on the budget available to the OT and the storage space available. Many of the books in the References and Further Reading give lists of useful toys.

Essential items for the playroom include:

- dolls' houses and dolls' house figures
- a sand tray
- modelling materials
- art materials
- construction toys
- puppets

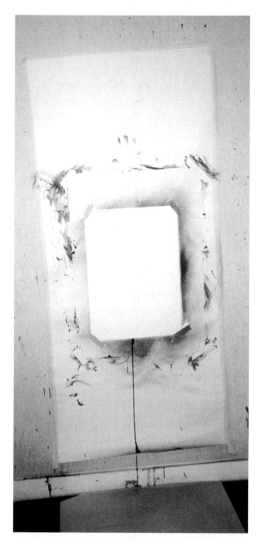

Figure 6.4 Area where messy regressive play is possible.

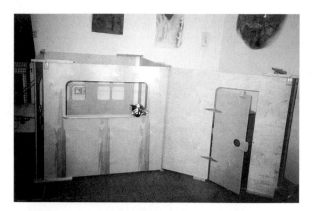

Figure 6.5 Multiple use structure.

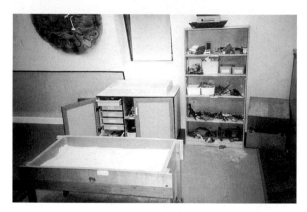

Figure 6.6 Sandtray and shelves.

- toys for regressive play
- large bean bags
- miniature animals and figures
- dressing up materials
- story books
- assorted games and soft balls.

An excellent list of sources of play materials and books can be found in the *Handbook of Play Therapy* (McMahon 1992).

Many play therapists are not able to operate in such good conditions, but if the room is the same and the equipment is in roughly the same places, the child will identify that place as special for therapy.

Preliminary meeting with the child and carers

This meeting may take place in a different room from the therapy room. It is preferable to use the room where the child will be having play therapy. This familiarises the room to the child before they come to therapy on their own. It also gives them permission from their parents to be there.

Some parents find it threatening to know that their child would be talking to a stranger about personal or family matters, and need to be reas-

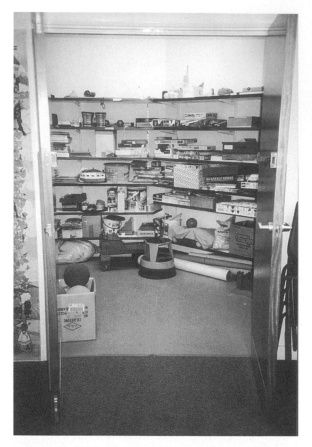

Figure 6.7 Walk-in cupboard.

sured about play therapy and how it will work for them. The initial meeting gives an opportunity to make dates for review, possibly about every four sessions, so that the parents are able to see the OT on their own to discuss the progress of the therapy and to voice any concerns. The content of the play therapy sessions would not be discussed, but an overview of progress given. Very anxious parents may need some sessions with another worker to run alongside the play therapy sessions.

During the meeting the child listens to what is being discussed, which helps to clarify the therapist's role for the child. Information is also gathered about ethnic, cultural and religious differences in beliefs, attitudes and behaviours which may need to be known to carry out the

therapy. This is especially important if you are dealing with a child who has experienced bereavement.

Care has to be taken not to become the counsellor for the parents during this initial interview. The OT will ask the parents why they are bringing their child for play therapy in order to clarify the reasons and possibly to get a list of behaviours. For example, the parents may say that the child is having nightmares or sleepwalking. They may want to list difficult behaviours the child is showing at home or at school, or both, and any other concerns. It is very important that this is not a wholly negative list of things that the child has done wrong, and it is useful to involve the child in the discussion to hear their point of view. The parents are also asked for the good points about the child so that the therapist observes the child's reaction to the positive comments the child hears about himself or herself. Younger children will probably be roaming around the playroom, using different items while the adults talk. Some children may react strongly to something that is being said by pounding a beanbag or throwing sand around the place. This may be responded to by the OT at the time or discussed at the first play therapy session.

A very clingy child may be invited to play with the parents, using some of the toys in the room to relieve anxiety. Observations of the child's reactions to being in the playroom with the parents may be used for future planning of play therapy sessions. Does the child join in with the conversation or ignore the parents? How do they react; are they clingy or inappropriately compliant or argumentative?

Ground rules for the use of the playroom are discussed with the child. The parents are usually as surprised as the child that it is acceptable to leave the room in a mess, to throw paint at a certain wall in the room or to punch a beanbag. The contrast between the playroom and the schoolroom or living room at home has to be made clear. The child gets to know it is permissible to express him or herself in whatever way feels comfortable within the constraint of certain rules, and that it is permissible to disclose and talk about issues that are private and confidential.

Accountability and confidentiality are to be agreed between the OT, referrer and/or other professionals or carers and the child so that boundaries are clear, and confusion and manipulation are avoided. Everyone is made aware, including the child, that if a matter of concern, for example abuse, is disclosed by the child, it will be shared with the appropriate professionals. The therapist maintains confidentiality about the details of the sessions, but may wish to explain to the carers and the child that the sessions will be discussed with their supervisor. There may be times when it is useful to be able to discuss the play therapy with the child's teacher or social worker, but permission from the parents and child should be obtained.

Practical details about the timing of the sessions, transportation and, especially for children, their way of asking to go to the lavatory and where it is need to be ascertained.

When children have been bereaved, it is useful to know whether they have been to the funeral or cremation and what took place at this time. When children have been sexually abused it may be necessary to know the child's terms for body parts and sexual acts, if it is possible to ask the carers during the meeting.

Carers need to be encouraged to dress the children in clothes that are easily washable and, if the child has to go to school straight afterwards, to provide a place where they can change back into school clothes. The therapist needs to be aware of whether the family is telling the school that the child is coming to play therapy or not. Some families prefer not to tell the school because they feel that the child will be stigmatised if it is known they attend the child and adolescent mental health service.

The way the decision is made for the sessions to end needs explanation. The child's point of view, as well as looking at the child's play and progress in the sessions, may give the therapist the view that the work is coming to an end. There will be feedback from the carers and also from other professionals who are involved with the family, and a decision will be made on the whole picture. The child needs to know that they will be informed about the progress of the therapy and will have time to prepare for the ending of the sessions. The child and the carers need to be confident of the key elements of the play therapy as being security and safety of the child with the therapist.

PLAY THERAPY ASSESSMENT

There is no right or wrong way to play; the process of playing is more important to the child than the outcome of that play (Fig. 6.8). It is therefore difficult to formalise play therapy assessments with a standardised administrative procedure unless this can allow for the surprising creativity of a child. An OT using a directive approach in play therapy assessment has to be ready to change to a non-directive approach in order to allow play to continue, rather than play becoming a task.

Test of playfulness

Anita Bundy (1997, p. 52), writing in *Play in Occupational Therapy for Children*, states: 'Unlike work and self care, the play activities in which individuals engage may matter less than whether the individual approaches those (and other) activities in a playful manner. It may be playfulness, rather than play activities that, when evaluated, provides therapists with the information they seek regarding their young client's development'. Bundy has developed a test of playfulness (TOP), which gives a framework for the systematic evaluation of playfulness in young children. Each child is observed for internal or external perception of control, intrinsic or extrinsic source of motivation, and free or not-free suspension of reality in order to give a playfulness profile.

Many non-standardised play therapy assessments are used, not only to assess the child's playfulness, but also to observe the child's verbal and non-verbal responses, their level of activity, concentration, distractibility, decision-making processes, ability to use play materials, interaction with the therapist and the process, form and extent of play. The OT will also be noting any indicators of perceptive or motor coordination problems that might not have been addressed.

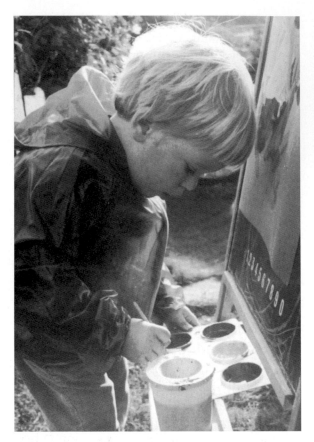

Figure 6.8   The process of playing is more important than the outcome of that play.

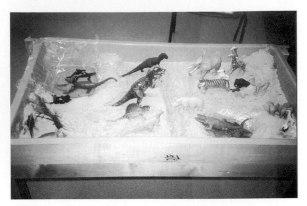

Figure 6.9   Sand world.

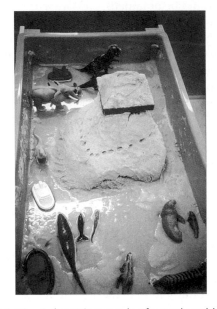

Figure 6.10   A dynamic example of a sand world.

Lowenfeld sand world technique

Margaret Lowenfeld developed the sand world techniques, which could be used as assessment and/or treatment, in which children were asked to construct a sand world in the sand tray. The tray had to be a specific size and coloured blue inside, and a large variety of miniature world material would be divided up in groups in small drawers in a cabinet to include figures of people, wild and domestic animals, houses, transportation, furniture, fences, trees and unstructured materials (e.g. pebbles). Lowenfeld saw the sand worlds as a way of expressing feelings and thoughts that may not make sense in the ordinary way. It was a way in which the children could describe to themselves and to the adult the nature of their experiences (Lowenfeld 1964). She devised a variety of scoring procedures, asking the child to explain their world to her and making no interpretations of her own. When this method is used in therapy, the sand worlds are done in a series that may be repetitive (Fig. 6.9), have external significance, or be what Lowenfeld called a 'dynamic example', which she thought could change the whole life picture of the child (Fig. 6.10).

This technique has been adapted by many different therapists; some ask the children to 'put themselves into' the sand world, and others ask the children to make up a story about what is happening in the sand world.

One Lowenfeld family therapist regularly uses a large sandpit for the whole family to build a 'world'. She observes each interaction, the toys and where they are placed, but remains a passive observer. Often these sessions are videotaped and shown to the family in later sessions to illustrate the family relationships being discussed. In one session worked this way with a family consisting of mother, father and 4-year-old son, the two adults became very engrossed in their play, creating a beautiful sand world without any relationship to what their child was trying to make in the sandpit. One parent even took one of the child's toys and used it in what he was doing, whilst the other erected a fence as a barrier to the child's corner of the tray. When the family saw the video, words were not needed to explain the child's low self-esteem.

Lowenfeld mosaic techniques

Lowenfeld also used a mosaic technique where the mosaics became a projective instrument (Figs 6.11 & 6.12). She believed that it was possible to gain a unique view of the person in action using this technique as an assessment tool, providing the therapist with a range of information about the child that differs significantly from the information provided by other tests.

Training is needed in Lowenfeld therapy to use her techniques for formal assessment. Her methods are well liked by many OTs who are using play therapy techniques because Lowenfeld's emphasis on observation, attention to detail, looking at the whole picture and using play as the treatment medium links well with the OT model.

Puppetry

Puppetry may be used as a tool in assessment. A wide range of puppets, representing realistic as

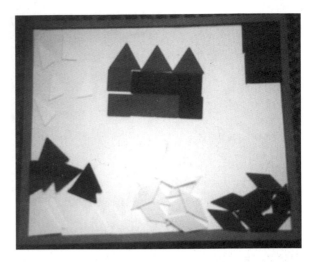

Figure 6.11 Example of a Lowenfeld mosaic.

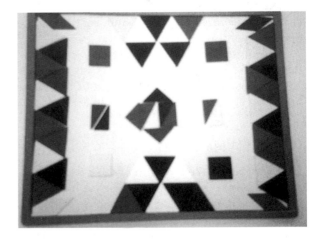

Figure 6.12 A Lowenfeld mosaic.

well as imaginary figures, is needed for the child to choose from (Fig. 6.13), as well as a construction that can be used as a puppet theatre. The child is asked to choose whatever puppets they like and to begin a story by introducing the puppets to the 'audience' (therapist). At the end of the play the child interprets the story to the therapist, who at that point may be taking the role of a reporter from the local paper.

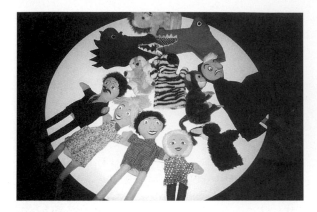

Figure 6.13   Puppets.

The content of the story, the characters chosen, and the way the child uses the characters and relates with them, are all helpful in learning about the child's world and how it is perceived by the child. Finding out who in the story the child would most like to be, and least like to be, can also be illuminating.

A disjointed, fragmented story may mirror how the child is feeling about him or herself. The characters chosen to help the child out of dilemmas are also a clue to the way forward in therapy.

Using dolls' houses

It is helpful to have two dolls' houses in the playroom, set apart so that the child who has moved house is able to reconstruct the move, indicating the people who moved too or stayed behind, and the new household established. Small dolls are used to represent the family members, and toy animals the family pets. The child may take on the roles of the different dolls used and speak for them or ask the therapist to join in, telling her what to say. In this way the child is often more able to verbalise feelings about the situation and where the confusions lie.

Another method used is to ask the child to set up one dolls' house as near to their own home as possible, to choose figures representing family members and the child, put them all to bed, and then get them up in the morning and run through a normal day or a particular day that is significant to the child. This gives a picture of the child's view of the home situation and where difficulties lie.

Family play assessment

One family play assessment involves using a number of planned exercises, in which even the youngest child in the family can take part, in order to observe the family dynamics (Blunden 1988). The OT does not take part in the activities, but observes the interactions. The family is asked to build a tower using 12 large wooden blocks. The therapist observes who directs the building, who builds the tower and who is passive, and takes no part. Does the family enjoy the task or get easily discouraged if the tower falls down? Who interacts with whom, and how? Other tasks, such as asking the family to sort a pack of playing cards into groups with a time limit, having a family discussion on their likes and dislikes, or planning a day out, assist in understanding the way the family functions.

GOALS AND OBJECTIVES OF PLAY THERAPY

Objectives of the play therapist are:

- to communicate with the child
- to understand the child's inner world and to effect changes in that world.

Katherine and David Geldard list four levels at which goals can be set. Level 1 goals are fundamental goals, level 2 goals are the parents' goals, level 3 goals are those formulated by the counsellor, and level 4 goals are the child's. All of the goals are important and have to be kept in focus during the therapeutic process. At various times during the process some goals need to have preference over others, and how this is achieved will be a responsibility of the therapist. Level I goals – fundamental goals – are globally applicable to all children in therapy and include the following (Geldard & Geldard 1997, p. 3):

- to enable the child to deal with painful emotional issues;
- to enable the child to achieve some level of congruence with regard to thoughts, emotions and behaviours;
- to enable the child to feel good about himself;
- to enable the child to accept her limitations and strengths and feel OK about them;
- to enable the child to change behaviours that have negative consequences;
- to enable the child to function comfortably and adaptatively within the external environment (for example at home and school);
- to maximise the opportunity for the child to pursue developmental milestones.

To achieve these goals it is important to give precedence to the child's goals whilst attending to the parents' and counsellor's goals. The child's goals are discovered as therapy proceeds. The parents' goals are set by the parents when they attend the initial interview, and they are usually based on the child's behaviours. Level 3 goals are formulated by the therapist. Therapists draw on information from their clinical experience, theoretical understanding of child psychiatry and their knowledge of current research to formulate their goals. These goals need to be reviewed continually during the course of therapy and may need to be amended as the therapy proceeds. Understanding the child's needs takes practice and experience.

NOTE-KEEPING AND REPORT WRITING

Note-keeping fulfils different functions and varies in the way it is done, according to the OT's way of working and the protocols in place in the work setting.

Some OTs may keep their own set of working notes and write summaries for the main case notes every four to six sessions. Others may write each session directly into the case notes where there is a section for each discipline involved with the family.

Reports need to be written to the referrers and may be requested by other professionals involved with the family. The OT will have to be clear about the issues of confidentiality, and written permission may have to be gained from the family to contact professionals outside the multidisciplinary team, for example teachers.

Working notes

These should be written straight after the play therapy session if possible. The notes should be dated, timed and signed, and consist of detailed recording of everything done and said by the child and play therapist in a chronological order. Many incidents that seem trivial or insignificant during the session may in later sessions be very important in understanding the process of therapy taking place.

Things to note include:

- the way the child separates from the carer in the waiting room and the child's approach to the play therapy session
- non-verbal communication by the child as well as the way the child moves around the room and approaches different activities within the play therapy
- feelings expressed by the child during the session and any links that are made to previous sessions.

The OT will also record their own feelings about the session, transference issues and issues to be followed up in subsequent sessions.

The importance of writing about one's work and reflecting on it has been discussed by Dee Walker (1985): 'Writing can help nurses to distance themselves from an experience and thus reflect it more objectively, to differentiate between what actually happened and what they think happened. Writing can help the individual to revisit an experience when perceptions about it may have changed. The pace of work or emotions may impede on the spot reflections but writing about it afterwards may prove even better'.

Many OTs find sketching parts of the therapy session a helpful way to record what happened. The sketches may include a sand world sequence, repetitive movements made by a child around the playroom, a sketch of the child's painting or clay work. Some OTs may take photos with a Polaroid camera to include in the notes. Alternative recording schedules are described in Janet West's (1994) book *Child Centred Play Therapy* on page 176, as are ways of recording group work (p. 179).

Report writing

Reports summarise the working notes and are usually written after every four to six play therapy sessions. The reports will also include factual information about the reason for referral, other professionals involved, date, times and length of play therapy sessions, and the method of play therapy being used. The process of intervention and significant scenes emerging from the play therapy will be recorded, together with a description of the play to illustrate the use the child is making of the sessions.

Review sessions with the child's carers should be recorded, as well as any discussions with other professionals involved with the family. The final report would also include a review of the child's problems, changes noted during therapy, reasons for ending the therapy, and recommendations for future work if this is appropriate. All reports and working notes should be dated and signed, and reference made to anybody receiving copies of the report. See Chapter 15 for the legal aspects of record-keeping.

ENDING THE THERAPY

There is never a true ending to any therapy since children only handle work based on their particular developmental level. Sometimes new symptoms emerge at new developmental stages.

A good rule of thumb is that the longer the period for which the child has had play therapy, the more preparation there needs to be for the ending of the sessions. The child needs to feel part of the decision to end the sessions, and time must be taken for the relationship to change between the child and the OT so that the child can express feelings about the end of therapy and gain confidence in being in control of the way therapy ends.

In the normal course of therapy the OT, together with the child and referrer, will have discussed the progress that has been achieved

and the end of the therapy will be planned over a few sessions. There are many ways of ending the sessions; some OTs may take photos of the playroom for the child to take away or give them something as a transitional object when they are moving from one form of therapy to another. Others send cards or presents or have a mini-party in the playroom at the last session.

An opportunity is given for the child to talk openly about their feelings as therapy is ending. It is helpful to keep all the child's artwork and ceramics until the last session to allow them to review the sessions and decide which items they want to keep and which to destroy. It is not unusual for the child to want to make a card or a picture in the last session to leave in the playroom.

Younger children may colour in a chart, which has representation of the last four sessions. This helps them to count down the sessions and then take the chart away with them at the last session.

Many therapists book a follow-up appointment 2–3 months later so that there is not a sharp cut-off in therapy for the children who have experienced many losses in their lives. Others send cards or letters on birthdays to show that the child is not forgotten.

Unplanned endings

There are situations when the child has suddenly moved away or cut off from therapy unexpectedly. In this case it is important for the OT to try to arrange a final session with the child and, if possible, to transfer the child to another play therapist within the new locality. It is important for the child to understand that it was not the OT who decided upon the therapy ending and that the therapist may want to write an ending letter to the child expressing this.

When the therapy is coming to an end, some children will raise new issues. The OT will have to decide whether these issues need to be dealt with as a continuation of therapy or after a break from therapy, or whether they are part of the child not feeling they have enough inner strength to make progress on their own. Many children referred for play therapy have undergone multiple separations. They need time to talk through their feelings about therapy ending in order to avoid feeling rejected again.

The process of ending therapy, particularly if the child has been in therapy for a long time, also has implications for the OT, who needs to facilitate the change from a therapeutic relationship to a real relationship with the child. Good supervision at this stage will help OTs to understand their own feelings and reactions (see Ch. 14).

The Therapist's Journey

Janet West, in her book *Child Centred Play Therapy*, says:

'Play therapists are encouraged to take responsibility for their own wellbeing in order to maintain themselves so that they can support a traumatised child. Workers who fail to care for their physical, spiritual, emotional and cognitive needs, both conscious and unconscious, are in danger of harming themselves and the children whom they strive to serve'.

So how do we do this? When faced with the inhumanity of abuse to little children who have witnessed and experienced things which are difficult to imagine and as play therapists listen to, accept, understand and feel something of what the child is conveying of these experiences, it is easy for the therapist to become emotionally drained and overwrought.

The therapist needs to understand the emotional effects of her work on herself and needs to seek help and supervision for her cases and know when to stop and rest. It is essential to have a life away from work to be creative and keep things in perspective.

A poem by Ulrich Schaffer to finish, called *The Completeness of this Child*.

The Completeness of this Child

I am amazed
at the completeness of this child:
nothing is missing
this is a person like I am.

There is a richness of emotion,
a struggling with the will,
a facing of anxiety,

abandonment in joy,
a life full of hope and failure,
of disappointment and joy,
a life not different from my own.

The doubts and fears of being loved or not
can hurt and kill at three or ten or thirty:
the danger is
that in looking back
we laugh at what we thought
when we were small,
and then transfer those laughs
to children in our life
who might be living at the limits of their lives.

The one who dies
at three or ten or thirty
must first of all be seen
with his own eyes.

I have to take more seriously
each phase of growth,
and learn to live inside the head
that feels and doubts and questions.

I have to remind myself
that to a child
life is just as big
as it is to me.

I think of Christ
taking a child,
putting it in the middle
and saying:
'Unless you turn
and become like children
you will never enter the kingdom of heaven.'

Again and again
I wonder what that means.

Ulrich Schaffer.

ACKNOWLEDGEMENTS

I would like to thank Local Health Partnership NHS Trust for their encouragement and express my thanks to Sylvia Mickleburgh for typing the manuscript.

REFERENCES

Alessandrini N A 1949 Play – a child's world. American Journal of Occupational Therapy 3:9–12
Axline V 1947 Play therapy. Churchill Livingstone, Edinburgh

Blunden P 1988 Diagnostic interview using family tasks. National Association of Paediatric Occupational Therapists' Newsletter Spring: 9–10

Bowlby J 1988 A secure base. Basic Books, New York

Bundy A C 1996 Play, possibilities, problems, paradoxes. National Association of Paediatric Occupational Therapists' Newletter Autumn:29

Bundy A C 1997 Play and playfulness: what to look for. In: Parham L D, Fazio L S (eds) Play in occupational therapy for children. Mosby, St Louis, ch 4, p 66

Cattanach A 1994 Play therapy – where the sky meets the underworld. Jessica Kingsley, London

Geldard K, Geldard D 1997 Counselling children – a practical introduction. Sage, London

Klein M 1932 Psychoanalysis of children. Hogarth Press, London

Lowenfeld M 1964 The non-verbal thinking of children and its place in psychotherapy. Waterlow, London

Lowenfeld M 1967 Play in childhood. Wiley, New York

McMahon L 1992 Handbook of play therapy. Routledge, London

Monson S 1995 The use of play in family therapy. National Association of Paediatric Occupational Therapists' Newsletter Summer: 23

O'Connor K J 1991 The play therapy primer. John Wiley, New York

Oaklander V 1978 Windows to our children. Real People Press, Moab, Utah

Rogers C 1951 Client-centred therapy. Houghton Mifflin, Boston

Schaffer U 1980 For the love of children. Lion Publishing, England, p 14

Sloves, Belinger-Peterlin K 1994 Time limited play therapy. In: Shaefer C E, O'Connor K J (eds) Handbook of play therapy – advances and innovations. Wiley, New York

Walker D 1985 Writing and reflections. In: Bond R et al (eds) Reflection: turning experience into learning. Kogan Page, London

West J 1994 Child centred play therapy. Edward Arnold, London

Winnicott D W 1971 Playing and reality. Tavistock, London

Yorke C 1982 Psychoanalytic psychology of normal development. Hogarth Press, London

FURTHER READING

Axline V 1964 Dibs: in search of self. Penguin, Harmondsworth, UK

Cattanach A 1992 Play therapy with abused children. Jessica Kingsley, London

Dwivedi K N (ed) 1993 Groupwork with children and adolescents. Jessica Kingsley, London

Gil E 1991 The healing power of play – working with abused children. Guilford Press, New York

Wilson K, Kendrick P, Ryan V 1992 Play therapy – a non-directive approach for children and adolescents. Baillière Tindall, London

Winicott D W 1980 The Piggle. An account of the psychoanalytic treatment of a little girl. Penguin, Harmondsworth, UK

7

Family therapy, systems theory and the Model of Human Occupation

Becky Durant

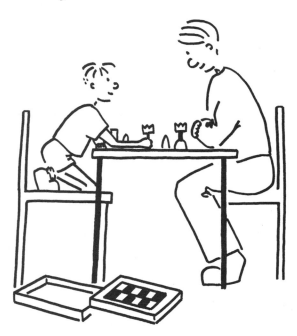

The problem is the child. The child has the problem. Change the child and the problem will go away. What would happen if we changed the problem? Would the child go away?

It is probably true to say that not so very many years ago most therapists' thinking was 'linear' and people gave children labels that reinforced their linear view that the child was the problem. This gave credence to the use of individual therapy, possibly non-directive play therapy in child and family settings. The task of these centres was to treat the child in order to get rid of the problem. This reductionistic approach remained prominent until the late 1970s, when there was a massive shift in thinking and a change of focus from a cause-and-effect model to a circular, systemic paradigm, probably influenced by early postmodernistic thinking. The primary focus of attention was no longer the child. Therapists began thinking differently about the problem, how it is created and how it can be resolved.

The family was seen as the 'system' and each family member was viewed as an equally important part of this system. Eventually the total context of the child was considered, and nowadays it is quite fashionable to view schools or neighbours or other family members as part of the system, and thus broaden the original idea of 'significant others'.

Indeed the word 'system' became very fashionable until the late 1980s when it gained two more letters and became 'systemic', and family therapy evolved again until the new name 'systemic therapy' appeared. Nowadays, both terms are used but describe different methods. However, systemic therapists have moved a long way from the application of general systems theory upon which the theory of family therapy is based.

The development of family therapy and the changes it has experienced can, in a way, be likened to the transition that happened in Spain between 1975 and 1992. This has been described as a period of evolution and not revolution. Franco died in his bed, no-one killed him and, following his death, a slow but relatively successful transition to democracy occurred in a country that had endured 30 years of dictatorship. There were relatively few battles on the way, apart from problems with ETA – EUSKADI TA ASKATASUNA (Basque Separatist Movement) – and a failed attempt to overthrow the government in November 1998. Things, seemingly, were allowed to happen and few challenged the existing PSOE (the Spanish Socialist Party).

Likewise, in family therapy very little scientific theory has proved or disproved theories or concepts, and family therapy has evolved and changed gradually over the past 20 years. Indeed 'systemic therapy' evolved from 'systems theory' but throughout its journey took on different names or descriptions. For example, for a while people became interested in 'structural family therapy', which differed from 'strategic' or 'behavioural' family therapy. There are many other examples of types of family therapy but all have their roots in systems theory.

Ideas, derived from the biologically based theories of Maturana & Varela (1972, 1988), have challenged therapists' certainty about objective reality and indeed about their objective judgements of others. Also the idea about change and the likelihood of being able to change others has led to the creation of thinking differently. Now there exists the possibility of questioning certain traditional theories and value systems. Together with this is the realisation that there can be many opinions and solutions which can be accorded equal status. The purpose of this chapter is to outline the changes in family therapy in the postmodern world and to consider the importance of systems theory in relation to family therapy and a particular model of occupational therapy.

WHAT IS A 'SYSTEM'?

The word system emerges all over the place in literature relating to family therapy, and so it deserves a definition. A system refers to any mixture of composed elements that interact and together constitute a whole with a purpose of function. Concepts relating to systems are applied to a very large range of different phenomena, for example a family system, the digestive system, the educational system. Each system shares universal properties and it may be useful to understand one type of system in order to make sense of another. People need to connect with others to experience responses and gain information which in turn leads to the development and support of the belief system they have about themselves.

Open systems theory was developed to explain and understand living phenomena. Many of its ideas stem from biology as it refers to all life forms. These systems are defined as dynamic and self-organising and interact continuously with other environments (von Bertalanffy 1968a, b).

Dynamic systems theory describes the way in which new states of organisation emerge spontaneously as a result of the flow of sufficient energy through systems. The components behave in ways that are impossible to predict by looking at their individual properties.

These ideas offer interesting similar and overlapping concepts and it is quite difficult to differentiate between them. Family therapy emerged using ideas from all these concepts and thus refers to all of them as 'systems theory'. Styles of therapy have changed as new concepts emerge. Many arose from the work of von Bertalanffy, the founder of general systems theory. There is a more detailed section on 'systems theory' and systems in a later section of this chapter.

POSTMODERNISM

Postmodern models of therapy highlight the clinician's role as non-hierarchical and stress the therapist as embedded in the same proces of social construction as are the individual and the family. In other words, 'there is fluidity of social interaction in the construction of meanings we assign to phenomena' (Pare 1995, p. 2). The therapist moves from an analyst who diagnoses a family dysfunction and then intervenes to correct it, to a participant observer of family interaction. Nowadays therapists have the benefit of being 'systems analysts' and 'postmodernists', and can probably incorporate both approaches at the same time. Therapy is fluid, the therapist's role is fluid, and the therapist can dance backwards and forwards from one way of being to another.

Goals are to perturb 'meaning' systems (Varela 1989). Many postmodern family therapists characterize their family therapy in new ways. For example, Anderson & Goolishan (1988) have described the role of the postmodern family therapist as a master 'conversationalist'.

So what exactly is postmodernism?

Originally postmodernism derived from the humanities and incorporated the critiques of 'modernity' from such diverse thinkers as Michel Foucault and Jean François Lyotard (Sarup 1993). They share an antiobjectivist, antifoundationalist stance to what is in the world to what we can know in the world. They question the idea that by applying reason and scientific methods we may come to know or even more closely guess at an objective reality. This idea may not sit very comfortably in the new world of evidence-based practice to which more and more occupational therapists are subscribing. How can one use a mixture of systemic ideas and postmodernism in a new world of scientific reasoning, audit and evaluation? Perhaps this is a subject to be addressed in another book.

In the postmodern world there is an emphasis on construction and context. The system is a context, a multiple context, with multiple realities, and leads to a radical departure from Enlightenment conceptions of the individual subject. Descartes proposed an abstract disembodied self ('I think therefore I am') and somehow this self transcends the body. This self is descibed as stable and essential from one context to the next. However, postmodern thinkers see the self as something that emerges from discourses; it actively incorporates, reproduces and evolves the contexts in which it participates (Sarup 1993).

Thus 'self' becomes a social accomplishment and not a social product. Personal identity is an activity rather than a thing, and individual experience cannot be separated from the contexts and conversations that give experience meaning and direction. In terms of general systems theory this is really no different, other than breaking down every action, every aspect of social interaction into minute parts and making sense of it in terms of greater but at the same time minute bits of the whole. Conversations become part of the system and meanings are constructed by parts of the system.

SYSTEMS THEORY

The word 'system' is a fashionable catchword. The notion has invaded all fields of science and has an active role in popular thinking. Its origins are complex. 'One aspect is the development from power engineering – that is, release of large amounts of energy as in steam or electric machines – to control engineering – which directs processes by low-power devices and has led to computers and automation' (von Bertalanffy 1968c).

Professions and jobs were given a new description (systems analysts, systems engineering), and now in therapy we have systems consultants and a derivative of the word system: systemic therapists. Technology is no longer thought of in terms of single machines, but in 'systems'.

Now we have missiles and space vehicles assembled from mechanical technology, but the relations of humans and machines also play an important part. We can no longer exclude the influence of political, social and economic problems. It is no longer a matter of numbers to be produced, but of a system to be planned and arranged. This has been called the Second Industrial Revolution and has been developing rapidly in the past few decades.

The developments have not been limited to industry; for instance, politicians frequently ask for application of the systems approach to overcome problems. In 1967, Canadian Prime Minister Manning wrote (Manning 1967):

An interrelationship exists between all elements and constituents of society. The essential factors in public problems, issues, policies, and programmes must always be considered and evaluated as interdependent components of a total system.

This theory was introduced by Ludwig von Bertalanffy (1968c), and his book *General Systems Theory* gives a very detailed account of its roots, development and usage. To understand the theory, it is interesting to know something about von Bertalanffy. The following is a summary of his background.

Ludwig von Bertalanffy began his professional career as a scientist when biology was involved in the mechanism–vitalism controversy. In other words, organisms were things that were organised and von Bertalanffy and other scientists were interested in finding out about it. He first talked about his idea of general systems theory way back in 1937, but at this time the idea of theory and theories in biology was not very popular and his ideas were not very well received. Indeed, his first publication did not appear until after the war.

It seems that a shift in thinking had then occurred which created an opportunity for von

Bertalanffy to play around with his ideas and declare them to his colleagues without fear of ridicule or rebuff. This may remind the reader of similar problems that Freud faced in introducing his ideas to a very rigid and critical audience.

However, model building and abstract thinking paved the way for general systems theory to be viewed as a separate entity and was no longer seen as the whim of an over-enthusiastic scientist.

General systems theory states that a system is a whole. Its components and attributes can only be understood as belonging to and as functions of the complete system. A system is an interdependent organisation in which the movements and expression of each of its components influence and are influenced by all the other parts. Thus a system is not simply a random collection of components.

In her book *Family Therapy*, Sue Walrond-Skinner (1976) uses the analogy of a game of chess to describe systems. She writes that it would not be very helpful to understand chess by looking at its pieces. You have to examine the game in detail and to work out how each piece affects the position and meaning of every other piece on the board. Likewise, you could view a bicycle in the same way. A bicycle is not a random collection of ball bearings, cogs, sprockets, chain and wheels. Each part has a very important role and is dependent on its neighbouring part to function and give meaning to the whole machine.

Systems theory emphasises the interrelationship between system components and between systems and supra-systems. Much emphasis is placed on communication or how the components within the system interact with one another. In systems theory, transactions are viewed as circular and as creating progressively more complex spirals of exchange. If you imagine a game of Chinese whispers, a secret message is passed from one person to another. Each time the message is received and passed on it may or may not remain the same. Usually, by the time the message gets back to its original owner it bears no resemblance to its beginning.

In this example of interaction, the message is modified or changed by its interaction with the various people along its course. This modification occurs in a circular process known as a 'feedback loop'. The last point in the cycle is fed back to the first point, indicating the dynamic nature of the whole process. In systems theory transactions are described as circular. These exchanges create more complicated spirals of exchange.

General systems theory proposes that we should recognise the world as a huge, interdependent, interconnected whole. This is not unlike Hippocrates' suggestion that the world is a circle without a beginning or an end. Everything in the world belongs to the larger whole and shares characteristics. Consequently general systems theory aims to identify and explain properties that are found across a range of possibilities (von Bertalanffy 1968a,b).

An example with a family would look something like this

A family comes to a child and family centre hoping for something to happen to change the situation they are now experiencing. Perhaps the family has suffered some form of breakdown in its feedback process, in its internal transactions with the other family members, or maybe with its external transactions with the world outside the family. Walrond-Skinner (1976) talks about the dysfunctional communication patterns in families as three types: blocked, displaced and damaged. With the first, we often see periods of silence, withdrawal and isolation, or even at times the really bizarre way of communicating through notes in order to write messages. In other words, transactions and communication between family members takes on a different form and the possibility of growth is reduced because there is a definite obstacle or block in the way, which makes feedback difficult. Silence and withdrawal are forms of communication but, if this has become the predominant form of communication over a long period of time, the opportunity to feedback or respond is in many ways locked.

The family secret

A less extreme example of blocked communication is the family 'secret'. Normally the only real secret is that nobody knows that everybody knows the secret. In this instance family members use extreme methods to protect the 'secret' and often collude with one another to do so. It could be that scapegoats appear as diversionary tactics to conceal the secret. In other words, parents or one parent will focus on one aspect of a child's behaviour for long periods or divert the topic of conversation back to a safe topic, maybe to avoid exposure of the secret. In the early days of family therapy the therapists used to wonder: 'What are you not talking about by talking about this?'

However, a cautionary note is worth mentioning here. In the early days of family therapy we were such keen people, full of new ideas and theories, that we would often inadvertently 'shut families down' by our over-enthusiastic approach. In our eternal quest for the secret, we often missed very relevant information and may have been disrespectful to our clients.

Displacement can sometimes occur through the eruption of symptoms. The actual symptom and the symptom-bearer become highly significant means of communication in the family and between its members. It could be that the symptom has become a displaced means of communicating something about the family. Some family therapists may be interested in the symptom that has been chosen, and who has chosen or been chosen to carry it. Some family therapists who use systems theory as their framework are interested in symptoms as interpersonal messages rather than intrapsychic meaning.

Communication processes can be severely damaged within the family. The 'double bind' is an important example of blocked communication. This idea was originally described by a group of research scientists in California. They proposed that every message is communicated at two levels: the report level, which is about information given, and the second level, which conveys a message about the information. For instance, a parent reacts to a child on hearing his C grades by saying, 'Well done' and at the same time looks disappointed or angry. In some way the parent is communicating that the first message ('well done') is at odds with the parent's posture and non-verbal communication. Sometimes this results in confusion and immobility; nobody says any more about the subject but both members remain dissatisfied.

The first level is usually conveyed in words and the second level is normally expressed through non-verbal gestures or facial expressions. For this type of communication to result in serious confusion, it has to take place within the context of a relationship that is important and has significance for both parties.

These are just some examples of the use of systems theory to explain what may be happening in a family. There are many other terms that have become fashionable, but over time have been redefined or replaced by something similar. Rather like the creation of the Spice Girls, presumably to fulfil a need, and when the need is superseded by something else they are reshaped as opposed to becoming totally redundant, which may be the desire of a few.

SYSTEMIC THERAPY

This type of thinking sits very well in postmodern society. I think it coincided with a great deal of soul-searching and critical thinking, especially amongst occupational therapists. Many became aware of the link between personal and professional development and personal and professional thinking. The notion of neutrality or suspending one's beliefs became important, but so did the recognition of these same beliefs. How can you suspend something unless you know what it is? Therapists suddenly rejoiced in the freedom given to exposing, declaring and talking about their prejudices. At last it was okay to say: 'I don't like . . . . , maybe . . . . , I'm not sure . . . . , can you help me sort out where I am coming from?'.

It became important to become in tune with yourself so that therapists could identify when they were being influenced by factors other than the material offered by the family. Everything became important and the gaps between events narrowed. This was scary for some, and exciting for others. But it can be fun to consider how everyday fashionable thinking may be influencing judgements.

In the postmodern world therapists started thinking about the process of change. When therapists worked as strategic family therapists, it was almost as if everything was much clearer. Things could be seen and solutions could be taught. The therapist was the expert who held the key to the solution. Effective problem-solving skills could be taught. For a more detailed description of structural and strategic family therapy, see Durant (1996).

Eventually in the new postmodern world, the notion of the 'expert' would have to go. The therapist no longer possesses the gift of superior knowledge that puts him or her in a superior position above that of the client. Thus, therapists began to question meaning and understanding. Is it really possible to understand our clients or only to understand the words they are using?

Nowadays, family therapists have a different role, from an analyst to a participant observer of family interaction. The goals are to 'perturb' meaning systems (Varela 1989). Hoffman (1992) described her role as a 'friendly editor'.

Family therapists have considered the problems of power and inequity within the cultures in which family therapy operates. At the same time there is the realisation of power attributed to therapists within social systems.

Second-order family therapists will continually recognise and acknowledge that their views are not objective or 'true' in any determinable way, but rather that they are constructed from the limited (but important) viewpoint of the therapist, and that clients should feel free to disagree.

From a personal standpoint, how easy is it for clients to disagree? Surely in a therapeutic setting the therapist's voice will always carry more weight? (Atkinson & Health 1990, p. 152)

So where does all this fit in with occupational therapy? The following is an attempt to look at occupational therapy in the postmodern world and is followed by a description of the Model of Human Occupation.

OCCUPATIONAL THERAPY IN POSTMODERNISM

It appears that occupational therapy training continues to be very broad, with still endless dialogues about its definition and arguments about its name. It has never allied itself to any particular universal truth system, other than that based on the theory of meaning in systems theory. So perhaps it is has always been postmodern.

In universities there is emphasis on the process model of teaching, as opposed to the product model. In therapy the move away from scientific objectivity means that the therapist's views, and gut feeling of situations and events, have greater importance. Lecturers and students collaborate to find out answers together: learning is a partnership. Perhaps the role of teacher as provider of knowledge, the expert, has changed. Likewise in therapy, occupational therapist and client enter into a shared world of exploration, creativity and discovery. Decisions are no longer based on grand theories but arise from their own experimentation and experientation.

This is surely being both brave and creative? People are given the freedom to move with the natural processes as they emerge. Truth becomes a process or a creation. It moves, it is dynamic, and is to be experienced, not observed.

However, the respectful 'being-with' position of some therapists can be perceived by others as almost an opting-out position. Worse still, the teacher or therapist no longer needs skills or knowledge: it is enough to be there to facilitate. Indeed some lecturers refer to themselves as facilitators and not as teachers. This fits in with the systemic idea of instructive interaction being an impossibility. This idea, originally explicated in biology by Maturana & Varela (1988), has been modified by systemic therapists. Basically it means that one person's actions cannot specify another person's response. The response depends on the person's structure, including physical, physiological, emotional and meaning-construing components. In other words, if you tell someone to do something, you cannot guarantee that they will do it. Similarly, if you give someone a piece of information, this does not mean that they will understand and interpret it in the same way as the person who gave it to them originally; neither does it mean they will remember it.

This idea has led to confusion with therapists – and maybe teachers too. Some have concluded that all action and intentionality on the part of teachers and therapists are useless. Others may have concluded that the therapist holds no responsibility for the reaction of the patient or student. This somewhat amoral stance could lead to the situation where teacher or therapist feels free to do nothing or anything, the assumption being that the student or patient will draw their own conclusions from the interaction.

Thus, if instructive interaction is impossible, then presumably one individual cannot exert power over another. Surely this is ludicrous as there are psychological and physical forces operating, as well as cultural influences, that may permit people to be dominated.

In the therapist–patient situation, the patient is likely to feel unhappy and uncomfortable and is coming to discuss private things with a stranger. The stranger (therapist) is on home territory and knows the rules, having played the therapist game many times before. It is a one-sided intimacy, in which the therapist is not going to expose personal problems.

The oversimplification of ideas has led some therapists and teachers to adopt a position that implies there can be total equivalence between the influence and responses of acts by various people in a system. So, when a frustrated student says, 'Please, just tell me the answer!' or a frustrated mother in therapy begs the therapist, 'What should I do when my son has a tantrum?', maybe we should just give a straight answer. After all, telling someone else what to do may open up a far wider range of possible responses with a less predictable outcome than if we 'worked through' all the possible scenarios with student or patient.

The following describes briefly one of the models of occupational therapy that shares some basic beliefs with the origins of family therapy and also recognises the importance of contexts.

MODEL OF HUMAN OCCUPATION

This model was first published in the 1980s by Kielhofner in the USA, and was subsequently modified in 1995. It seeks to explain the occupational behaviour of humans. Its origin is interesting because, according to Sally Feaver (1995, p. 364), 'The model was devised in response to a perceived need for occupational therapists to have a unifying structure for all practice fields'. What does this really mean and what are the implications?

The model itself hints at a need to create a model as a way of solving a problem amongst professionals as opposed to a need to understand our clients' problems more clearly. However, as a consequence, it is a useful way of explaining the occupational behaviour of humans. As all behaviour is 'occupational' in this model, this type of behaviour refers to behaviour with which the occupational therapist is concerned and defined as:

An activity in which persons engage during most of their waking time: it includes activities which are playful, restful, serious and productive. These work, play and daily living activities are carried out by individuals in their own unique ways based on their belief and preferences, the kinds of experiences they have had, their environments and the specific patterns of behaviors that they require over time. (Kielhofner 1985)

The model uses systems theory to conceptualise the human in much the same way as family therapists used systems theory to conceptualise the family. According to Feaver (1995, p. 364): 'The model conceptualises the human as a dynamic system which both affects and is affected by the environment.' The internal part of the system has three components:

1. Volition – this chooses and initiates action
2. Habituation – a subsystem that organises behaviour
3. Performance – a subsystem that contains the skills necessary to carry out the action.

The environment is viewed as objects, people and culture, which is assessed to determine whether or not it suppresses or illuminates a person's action. The process of intervention requires the assessment of all the subsystems. (The reader is advised to read Kielhofner (1995) for further explanation.)

Similarly, family therapists have described families as a dynamic system constantly changing

and affected by the environment. The family is the whole and comprises its component parts – the individuals within the family. The character of the family is a product of the characteristics of its component parts and how they react and interact with one another and, of course, the environment. Each part influences and is influenced by the other.

Both models are based on the idea of systems being open; the environment is seen as people, objects and culture. Family therapy models today probably overlap with the OT model with respect to the volitional subsystem. According to Kielhofner this section concerns itself with people's beliefs in themselves and their abilities, and the expectancy of success and failure in managing their own life.

Intervention would require an assessment of this subsystem and others to determine deficits and therefore to choose appropriate intervention, designed to minimise the effect of the disability or deficit upon a persons ability to perform. (Feaver 1995, p. 364)

This is reminiscent of therapist's references to families as dysfunctional. This term is seldom used nowadays in the world of family therapy because the concept of a 'functional family' has disappeared along with the therapist's ability to assess and prescribe.

However, as mentioned above, there are some similarities with the volitional subsystem as family therapists often make it their business to look at and identify belief systems. In family therapy it is considered as important for the therapist to look at his or her beliefs as it is for the patients to do so. Unless occupational therapists are working as family or systemic therapists, the author is unsure how this concept fits into the occupational therapy world. Do occupational therapists consider the origin of their views and expose them along with their biases and prejudices? Do they consider their professional and personal development to play an equal role in their beliefs as their cultural and familial backgrounds? Are therapists able to identify those times when they are being influenced by factors outside the therapy environment?

It is very hard to find a common language for family and systemic therapy as it grew from the work of several people. It has developed and changed direction, and many many people have published articles about new ideas and concepts.

New terminology has emerged and the field of family therapy is constantly being ploughed and reseeded. Systemic therapy has been influenced by sociology, anthropology and social psychology. Ideas change very quickly: as soon as one model is proposed another emerges. This mercurial quality of therapy can be very unnerving for the cautious – but exciting and challenging for the reckless.

First published 20 years ago, the Model of Human Occupation (Kielhofner & Burke 1980) was the first occupational therapy model to incorporate ideas from systems theory. A new second edition (Kielhofner 1995) contained changes and refinements that reflect new interdisciplinary theory, research findings and insights encountered in practice. It is curious that no-one other than Kielhofner has refined these ideas, unlike the world of family therapy where several people have contributed, developed or changed the original concepts. In the current family therapy journals there are constant articles challenging people's views, and lively debates about the meaning of words.

Many occupational therapists have published articles about occupational therapy models and have described the meaning or application of the model to particular settings (Atkinson 1995, Feaver 1995). Few have developed these ideas further or developed new ones. In the absence of lively discussion, there can be no debate.

CONCLUSION

Family therapy is, by nature, very specific and focuses on families; its theory is useful to a variety of professions. The occupational therapy model may be relevant only to its own profession. Occupational therapy focuses on techniques used with everyone – single people, children, the elderly – and not just families. Its usage is broader.

Family therapy came to the fore at a time when the family was apparently changing. The organisation and function of the family was no longer the same, and may have been threatened with disintegration or obsolescence. The increase in divorce and reconstituted families, and the acceptance of non-heterosexual or non-child-bearing structures within society's definition of the family, may offer greater flexibility. So the period of great change in family life also corresponds to the period of development of family therapy.

Occupational therapy training is very broad and does not necessarily ally itself to any particular universal truth, so it is hardly surprising that few ideas and beliefs emerge relating specifically to occupational therapy. Perhaps this reflects a true postmodern approach, as occupational therapists assume a flexible stance, dancing in and out of many different models that relate to therapy. They have the flexibility to work in a truly eclectic way. With less emphasis on objective reality, greater credence is offered to the occupational therapist's subjective interpretation of situations. A postmodernist recognises human experience and the importance of subjectivity. Intuition is afforded greater respect. Occupational therapists are able to adjust their actions and responses to meet the needs of each individual or family, and in turn become less self-conscious about valuing the subjective.

The wealth of literature on family therapy and systemic therapy provides an extraordinary academic presence, but it is occupational therapy that is established as a university subject. If we look back in 10 or 20 years' time, will we see current family therapy, systemic or occupational therapy theories as fitting in such a way into the maintenance of a particular social order? Will family therapy exist as a subject or profession taught in isolation at universities?

Have ideas generally developed as part of the changing world order? Why was it that the stance of the Model of Human Occupation took 15 years to be modified, whilst other similar ideas are constantly changing?

REFERENCES

Anderson H, Goolishan H A 1988 Human systems as linguistic systems: preliminary and evolving ideas about

is an instrument of research into the patient's unconscious' and is 'the most dynamic way in which his patient's voice reaches him' (Heimann 1950, p. 82). The study of projective identification can help us to understand how this happens.

Projective identification

Projective identification is a term that was introduced by Melanie Klein in 1946. Melanie Klein discussed it as a mechanism of defence in order to rid oneself of overwhelming anxiety. Bion (1962a) has, as was discussed in the section on the mother–infant relationship, drawn our attention to the use of projective identification as an earliest form of communication in normal development.

Projective identification is the mechanism whereby parts of the self are split off and projected on to the other person, who in turn identifies with the projected parts. The person projecting feels at one with the object of the projection. The projected feelings can then be reinternalized by the projector, after having been psychologically processed by the recipient (Ogden 1979). There are clear links here between Bion's concept of the mother's role in making distress tolerable for the baby, so that the baby can reinternalize the experience in a modified form. In therapy, the therapist often needs to hold on to the projected parts for long periods and gradually, over time, help the patient to 'take back' the split off parts. This requires therapists to be open to and aware of their own feelings in the therapeutic situation, and links in with the previous discussion of the need for a mental space in therapists' minds.

A central aspect of projective identification is the controlling of another person from within, by putting part of oneself into that person. A common scenario in child therapy that can helpfully be understood in these terms is when a child sets up role-play situations whereby the child is the powerful adult and the therapist is asked to take on the role of the helpless and persecuted child (Melzer 1967).

A further example of projective identification is when the child wishes to play a game and, after agreeing on a set of rules, keeps changing the rules, so that the child is constantly at an advantage and the therapist feels unable to get anything right, as the goalposts keep changing. In a behavioural way, the therapist may enter into a discussion about rules. From a psychodynamic perspective, however, this situation offers an opportunity to think with the child about what it feels like to have the goalposts constantly changing and also about the importance for the child to be in control at all cost. The situation offers to the therapist, if she is open to receive it, a hint of how the child experiences its world.

Ogden (1979) commented that the main therapeutic value may lie in the process of therapists making themselves available to receive patients' projections. It is important for therapists to take note when they find themselves feeling and reacting out of character with their normal mode of being. They may at these times be identifying with projections of the patient. They may feel restless, bored or sleepy, or perhaps useless or unable to get anything right. Although this may be because they are having a bad day, it is more likely that these feelings are linked with feelings that the patient is unconsciously conveying. If noted in this way, these feelings become important in the therapist's understanding of the child's communications.

Splitting

Splitting in the therapeutic setting refers to the splitting or separating off of unwanted internal experiences and feelings in order to keep them apart from good experiences and thereby protect the personality from overwhelming anxiety, or from a sense of being contaminated by these bad experiences. This section also considers the wider aspects of fragmentation and integration of the human mind, which is closely linked with the child's development of a sense of self (see Box 8.5).

The following example from Tanya's middle phase in therapy demonstrates this.

Children frequently introduce splitting into their play, both in therapy and otherwise. Play symbols are divided into goodies and baddies, boundaries are erected to keep dangers out or to stop dangers from escaping, to create safety. At

Box 8.5 Case study

Tanya had a need to keep her therapy and her external life completely separate. She perceived her therapy as somewhere where she dealt with painful issues from the past, including her abuse. Linked with the abuse were feelings of disgust, contamination, guilt, anger and extreme badness. Tanya felt she had to protect her external life, where she was coping reasonably well, from the impact of her past. This led her to react with extreme distress to any attempt by anyone to make links between the two. Seemingly benign questions from her foster mother about how she got on today in therapy, or from her therapist, following a Christmas break, about how her Christmas had been, would cause Tanya to tell them to shut up or she could not continue coming for therapy. At that stage she needed to keep her experiences separate – to do otherwise felt life threatening. The aim of therapy would be for Tanya gradually, over time, to begin to integrate these experiences in a safe setting. She needed to grasp emotionally that, although what had happened to her was bad, it did not make her a bad person and that the abuse was but one of many experiences that made her the person she was.

times the boundaries are effective, at other times not. Play materials such as miniature people, wild and farm animals, walls and fences, as well as a sand pit, offer the flexibility for the child to explore issues to do with splitting, keeping apart and bringing together.

Judy Shuttleworth (1989), in the book *Closely Observed Infants*, considers that 'Melanie Klein's work chiefly centred on the processes within the internal world which lead to (a) the development of a sense of a whole person (both self and other); (b) an awareness of being engaged in a relationship between whole persons; and (c) the capacity for symbol formation . . .' which underlies the wish to communicate with others. 'Klein used a model for understanding these processes involving the development of two types of emotional experience. She named them the paranoid-schizoid and depressive positions. They refer to perceptually and emotionally fragmented and to integrated states of mind respectively. They are *positions* rather than *stages* . . .' because they 'alternate throughout life as the individual copes with external and internal pressures which impinge on him' (Shuttleworth 1989, pp. 40–41).

In the paranoid-schizoid position the individual is unable to perceive the other person or themselves as a whole person and relates to part-objects only (compare this with the young infant perceiving his mother as part-objects controlled by him). The individual is therefore able to control the limited set of feelings he allows himself to experience rather than encompassing the full range of feelings engendered by the relationship in the depressive position, including disappointments and loss (Shuttleworth 1989).

As a therapist one is frequently witness to children struggling with issues to do with fragmentation and integration in very concrete ways (see Box 8.6).

Box 8.6 Case study

Polly, aged 11, had experienced several care placements and was yet again awaiting a new family, with the promise of permanency. According to her social worker, Polly was unable to talk about any of her experiences. During her first therapy session she was immediately attracted to a box containing several simple jigsaws. After tipping them all out on the floor and mixing the pieces together, she indicated to the therapist that they all needed to be sorted out. Whilst jointly engaged in the task of sorting this great muddle and fitting the pieces into whole pictures, the therapist talked to Polly about the great muddle that was her life and of how difficult it would be to sort out the parts so that any sense could be made of it. This led to Polly beginning to talk about missing people in previous foster families and her previous social worker. In subsequent sessions she needed to repeat the same activity time and time again as it seemed to represent something very real for her about the fragmented nature of her life and about her need to link the parts.

The example of Thomas (Box 8.7) illustrates the movement from the paranoid-schizoid position to the depressive position in one session.

Box 8.7 Case study

Thomas, aged 5, had been rejected by his natural parents and was awaiting the 'special family' who would be his 'forever family'. He was at the time fostered by a couple with whom he had formed a deep attachment. He would have wished nothing more than to be claimed 'forever' by this family, but he knew this would not happen.

In his sessions, Thomas was wild. There was a sense that he used activity to fend off feelings and to stop himself from thinking. During this particular session, he ran around the room to begin with, not settling to anything. He eventually settled to build a model out of 'stickle bricks'. When he was finished, he threw the model towards the ceiling and it crashed down on the floor, breaking into tiny pieces. Thomas looked at the pieces with despair and threw himself on the floor into a fetal position and sobbed: 'It's no good, I can never build it up again, it's all broken and it will never be alright again'.

Thomas had shifted from a position in which his behaviour was restless and fragmented to one where he was painfully in touch with real feelings of grief and disappointment. At that time, the role of the therapist was to stay with him in his grief by quietly acknowledging his feelings, rather than, for example, consoling him and suggesting that the model could be fixed again. This demands that the therapist bear the painful feelings that Thomas has conveyed. Thomas's use of activity leads to a more detailed consideration of this below.

Function of activity in the context of the relationship

The concept of activity is central to any occupational therapist. The child's natural activity is play. Winnicott (1971, p. 53) states that in playing, and perhaps only in playing, is the child or the adult free to be creative. Not all play activity is creative or therapeutic. Activity that looks like play may be the child keeping busy, in order to avoid thinking or knowing about that which is too difficult. Bion (1962a) explored the functions of true creativity, with the emotional experience of trying to know the self and others on the one hand, and of activity that is empty and meaningless on the other. He called these functions K (for knowing) and minus K.

Fantasy is an integral part of a child's play. Again, at times, fantasy can be used to hide from reality, instead of as a means to explore internal and external reality in a creative way. The author has had the opportunity to treat some children who were adopted from Eastern European orphanages in their second year of life. In their early years they were deprived of both meaningful human contact and of sensory stimuli. These children developed a fantasy world that was absorbed from popular culture, such as television cartoons or comics, that had no anchorage in the

real world. The children had little sense of themselves in the context of their external world, but would see themselves as players in their escapist fantasy world. They could not differentiate between fact and fiction. One little girl would draw cartoon characters endlessly, but reacted with confusion and terror if asked to draw a picture of herself. She said that her face was not really her face, it was a mask to hide someone scary and scared inside. She had made fantasy and activity her mask. She needed to be helped gradually to be in touch with very basic feelings to begin with and to build on these. Her adoptive parents needed help in seeing that not all fantasy is healthy and to accept that she needed specialist help, in addition to the love they could give her.

The author was confronted with these questions in a very different and challenging way when she was asked to see Ben, aged $2\frac{1}{2}$ years (Box 8.8).

Box 8.8 Case study

Ben, following a car crash, was paralysed from the neck down and presented with nightmares, tearfulness and unwillingness to eat. Although Ben had lost his mobility and therefore most of his capacity for physical activity, he was nevertheless able to play in a symbolical way, directing the therapist to manipulate miniature figures. In this way he seemed to explore issues to do with the crash, with death, with illness and with the fact that he would not be made better or mended. The helplessness felt by the therapist about how to be able to help Ben was taken care of: he kept her busy – until some weeks later when he trusted her enough not to want to play, or draw or talk. The inactivity was terrifyingly painful as in it was contained the impact of the awfulness of what had happened. The aim of therapy became to provide for Ben a space and a time when he did not need to take care of anyone or to protect anyone from their helplessness by his charm and by keeping them busy. His use of activity thereafter became less constant, more chaotic and the themes were much more difficult to make sense of. But there was a feeling that maybe it was there for him rather than for anyone else.

CONCLUSION

This chapter has sought to introduce the reader to the psychodynamic way of thinking about human communication. It is hoped that the ordinariness of these theories has been demonstrated in combination with their contribution to the understanding of highly complex dynamics and behaviour.

Psychodynamic theories span the whole life cycle. The way the infant experiences his world will have a crucial effect on the emotional health and personality development of the individual. Patterns in early relationships are often repeated unconsciously throughout life. The ability of the mother to hold her infant in mind and to provide for him within the love and affection of her 'reverie' will allow the baby gradually to develop his own sense of self, essential for eventual separation from the mother and for the ability to form and maintain subsequent reciprocal relationships.

Psychodynamic theories offer a view on life and also a therapeutic technique. In learning about them, the value of observation cannot be underestimated. Observing a baby in his home or an older child in the nursery or school offers an opportunity to think in a meaningful way about a child's communications without having to provide a response. In therapy, to the observation and thinking is added the therapist's responses.

Psychodynamically oriented therapy tends to be long term and therefore comparatively expensive. It needs to be reserved for the children and young people with the most complex needs, for whom short-term therapeutic measures are not effective and for whom therapy is not a luxury but a life-line. Today's push for evidence-based practice offers a real challenge for those practising in this field. Evaluation and research are therefore priorities if we are to develop our future practice on the basis of a well understood conceptual framework of psychodynamic theory.

REFERENCES

Axline V M 1989 Play therapy, 2nd edn. Churchill Livingstone, Edinburgh
Bick E 1968 The experience of the skin in early object-relations. International Journal of Psycho-analysis 49:484–486
Bion W R 1962a A theory of thinking. International Journal of Psycho-analysis 43:306–310
Bion W R 1962b Learning from experience. Heinemann, London
Copley B, Forrayan B 1987 Therapeutic work with children and young people. Robert Royce, London

Heimann P 1950 On counter-transference. International Journal of Psycho-analysis 31:81–84
Hoxter S 1977 Play and communication. In: Boston M, Daws D (eds) The child psychotherapist and problems of young people. Wildwood House, London, ch 10, p 202
Hunter M 1993 The emotional needs of children in care – an overview. Association of Child Psychology and Psychiatry Review and Newsletter 15(5):214–218
Isaacs Elmhirst S 1988 The Kleinian setting for child analysis. International Review of Psycho-analysis 15:5–12
Klein M 1946 Notes on some schizoid mechanisms. In: Money-Kyrle P E (ed) 1975 The writings of Melanie Klein, vol. III, Hogarth, London, pp 1–25
Lanyado M 1991 On creating a therapeutic space. Journal of Social Work Practice 5:1
Melzer D 1967 The psycho-analytical process. Clunie Press, Perthshire, Scotland
Ogden T 1979 On projective identification. International Journal of Psycho-analysis 60:357–373
Reber A 1995 Dictionary of psychology, 2nd edn. Penguin, London
Segal H 1988 Introduction to the work of Melanie Klein. Karnac, London
Shuttleworth J 1989 Psychoanalytic theory and infant development. In: Miller M, Rustin M, Rustin M, Shuttleworth J (eds) Closely observed infants. Duckworth, London, ch 2, p 22
Sinason V 1992 Mental handicap and the human condition. Free Association Books, London
Telford R, Ainscough K 1995 Non-directive play therapy and psychodynamic theory: never the twain shall meet? British Journal of Occupational Therapy 58(5):201–203
Winnicott D W 1960a The theory of the parent–infant relationship. Collected papers: through paediatrics to psycho-analysis. Tavistock Publications, London
Winnicott D W 1960b Ego distortion in terms of true and false self. Collected papers: through paediatrics to psycho-analysis. Tavistock Publications, London
Winnicott D W 1971 Playing and reality. Tavistock Publications, London.

FURTHER READING

Alvarez A 1992 Live company: psychoanalytic psychotherapy with autistic, borderline, deprived and abused children. Routledge, London

Axline V 1964 Dibs: in search of self. Penguin, Harmondsworth, UK

Boston M, Szur R (eds) 1983 Psychotherapy with severely deprived children. Routledge, London

Copley B 1993 The world of adolescence: literature, society and psychoanalytic psychotherapy. Free Association Books, London

Judd D 1989 Give sorrow words: working with a dying child. Free Association Books, London

Kaplan C, Telford R 1998 The butterfly children: an account of non-directive psychotherapy. Churchill Livingstone, Edinburgh

Lanyado M, Horne A (eds) 1999 The handbook of child and adolescent psychotherapy. Routledge, London

O'Shaughnessy E 1981 A commemorative essay on W R Bion's theory of thinking. Journal of Child Psychotherapy 7(2):181–189

Rustin M, Rhode M, Dubinsky A, Dubinsky H (eds) 1997 Psychotic states in children. Duckworth, London

Rustin M, Quagliata E 2000 Assessment in child psychotherapy. Duckworth, London

Stern D N 1985 The interpersonal world of the infant: a view from psychoanalysis and developmental psychology. Basic Books, New York

Symington J, Symington N 1996 The clinical thinking of Wilfred Bion. Routledge, London

Waddell M 1998 Inside lives. Psychoanalysis and the growth of personality. Duckworth, London

Wieland S 1997 Hearing the internal trauma: working with children and adolescents who have been sexually abused. Sage Publications, London

Occupational therapy appropriate to age

SECTION CONTENTS

Working with children is very different from the treatment of adults, as the therapeutic intervention must be appropriate to the developmental level of the child. The treatment of infants and very young children, described by Carol Hardy in Chapter 9, is concerned with effecting change predominantly in the parent–child relationship. Therapy with primary school children requires the involvement of parent/carers, but some interventions may be directed to the child, as outlined by Karin Prior in Chapter 10. Anna Flanigan introduces the challenge and rewards of working with adolescents in Chapter 11.

9

Infants and young children

Carol Hardy

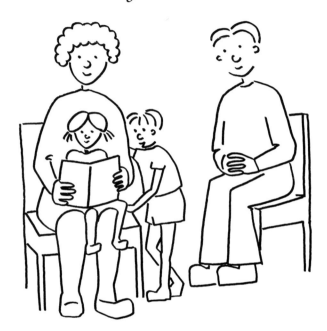

This title is chosen rather than the frequently
used description 'preschool' to reflect more of the
individual quality of this period in an infant and
toddler's life. They are not merely waiting to go

to school, but are in a position to make their first acquaintance with the 'outside world'. For the first few years of life this is mediated through the relationship and care they experience with their parents and/or primary care-givers. The richness of experience an infant and young child finds in a family where, more often than not, their needs are met for physical, emotional, social, communicative and playful interactions with a significant other should not be underestimated.

Child development research in the past 30 years has highlighted the fundamental importance of the relationship between parent and child, this being the place where an infant's mental and physical life is nurtured and developed (Brazelton et al 1991, Stern 1977, Trevarthen 1980). Detailed studies have shown the sensitivity a young infant brings to the contact with their primary carer and that it is in this interpersonal environment that mental life begins, in contrast to the assumptions underlying the work of previous child development researchers, who put a greater onus on the infant or child's interest and interaction with physical objects and specific skill-learning. Recent research shows the infants have an inborn interest and wish to connect with other human beings in order to make sense of themselves and their world (Brazelton 1991).

What use can we make of this to inform our practice in order to make a sufficiently sophisticated assessment of a young child's difficulties? It is useful to keep in mind Donald Winnicott's frequently quoted statement: 'There is no such thing as a baby' (Winnicott 1952, p. 99), to remind ourselves of the reality that a young child or infant is not functioning in this world in an independent fashion. Rather they are part of a dyadic relationship crucial at this stage more than at any other to keep them alive (see Ch. 5). It is therefore important that the nature of a young child's difficulties is understood in the context of the relationship with their parent(s). In many ways this can easily be understood by occupational therapists who have learned and comprehend the crucial link between an individual's function and their social environment.

UNIQUE QUALITIES OF 0–5 YEARS

What is the unique environment of an infant or young child? What is the purpose of it initially being so centred around the contact with one or two primary carers?

Intrauterine and pregnancy research (Piontelli 1992) indicate prebirth attachments developing. The infant's inborn predisposition to connect with its mother and father, is seen in early interpersonal awareness and specific actions towards the parents. For example, by 7 days babies will reliably turn their heads towards the smell of their own mother's breast pads and at 3 weeks the baby shows recognition of and a distinctive response to the mother's face (Brazelton & Cramer 1991).

Central to parenting is the individual 'fit' between parent and child. This 'fit' combines the general observations we can make about parents' qualities and skills with the individual characteristics the infant brings to the encounter (e.g. sensitive or 'laidback'). The 'fit' at any one time comprises how each side of the dyad meets together in an interactive relationship. It is in the space between parent and child that we see how negotiations and adaptations are made to one another, in a continual process of mutual influence and regulation (Brazelton et al 1974, Stern 1977, 1985, Trevarthen 1980).

In the early weeks and months there is predominantly a need on the infant's part to have parent(s) make adaptations to the infant. In order to do this the parent needs to understand what the infant needs, and how to organise their external environment (i.e. routines) and regulate the infant's internal environment (i.e. physiological and emotional states). At this stage the infant's capacity for self-regulation is limited, although some is present, for example gaze avoidance, muscular tension, hand to mouth. This is a crucial time for the infant's needs to be understood and met by others, as it is also the period in which they have the least ability to make their needs known. This preverbal time for a parent and child is extremely challenging and, although there is rich communication on one level, there is a necessity for the parent to be able to think from the infant's point of view (Winnicott 1986). The parents must use not only their cognitive abilities but also their emotional responses to understand what it is the infant is feeling and needing, and they need to be able to respond to the infant, regardless of their own needs and preferences at times.

The concept of 'containment' is a useful one to consider at this and later stages of life, as it combines both the sensitivity to the child's feelings by the parent and also the parent's ability to think around the emotional information they receive, adding their own perspective without losing the child's. An example of a 'containing' response may be when an infant becomes fretful and restless during a playtime with parent. The parent takes note of this, puts their own playfulness on hold for a few moments, and uses a calming voice to acknowledge the baby's agitation, thereby helping them to move on from this state and calm down. An 'uncontaining' action in the same situation would be, in response to the baby's fretting, that the parent withdraws from interacting with the baby and becomes an observer, thus leaving the infant to feel the full force of its distress alone. Another would be to respond to the baby with overt criticism and anger so the baby has to process its own negative feelings plus those of its parents (see Ch. 8 for further details on containment).

These are rather stark examples and in ordinary life no parent can always respond in a 'containing' way to all the infant's communications. If the greater number of responses is sympathetic, the infant will internalise an available figure. Tronick (1989) points out it is reparation of interactive failures (requiring initiation by the parent in the first years of life) that needs to occur in order for negative experiences, more often than not, to be resolved. Stern (1985) has described similar processes in his concepts of emotional attunement and misattunement. This experience of being helped to tolerate and overcome frustration will be a significant factor in how older children face problematic tasks and situations and try to resolve them (Tronick & Weinberg 1997).

Subtle change occurs in the developing infant and their relationships to others. The balance shifts gradually between the parent taking almost full responsibility, to the baby taking greater control of both its internal state, for example being able to wait a few moments longer for something, and the external environment. Knowing when to intervene and when to stand back in order to facilitate the child's development is highly skilful and is dependent on parental sensitivity and the dyadic 'fit'. When the balance between parent and child is well established and there is a smooth, rhythmic nature to the interaction, 'blips' may arise but are soon overcome. Much of the complexity of interaction in these circumstances goes unnoticed as it has an ongoing smooth quality.

It is important to keep in mind what are the essential ingredients for things to go well when we try to understand the difficulties between young children and their parents. It is often the absence of areas of regulation, communication, facilitation and negotiation between parent and child that is the key to understanding how the more overt interaction seems to be going awry, causing unhappiness for child and parent alike.

ROLE OR POSITION OF THE THERAPIST

What position does the occupational therapist or worker take in relation to the young child and their family? Let us consider first some of the particular qualities of this age group, which may have an effect on what stance we take in trying to engage the referred child and family. Also to be considered is the broad context in which these children and families are seeking help, a context that is related to some breakdown in family functioning, since the parents have not been able to resolve the issues within the immediate family, their extended family or community health environment. Seeking help can be acutely felt by many parents as their sole failure, especially if the young child has not yet started full-time education, at which point parents may attribute difficulties to the school environment.

For many families with children aged 0–5 years seeking help from child and adolescent mental health services (CAMHS) there may be no clear event or time at which the difficulties began with the child. This can make parents feel more exposed and vulnerable about the part they have played in their child's problems, and reinforce their feelings of disappointment in the way things have turned out. Some parents will be particularly driven to find a reason that is outside their arena. The most common example is to place the difficulties at the child's door, by suggesting genetics or specific organic conditions as an explanation. As these parents may also feel guilty as well as having such coping strategies they do require empathy, rather than over-reassurance, during the assessment period.

Taking an attachment theory framework (see Ch. 5) to examine a context in which an infant or young child is developing highlights the inevitability of a strong attachment to one to two primary attachment figures. This presents a challenge to the therapist. The difficulty lies in finding a balance between engaging the child and parent, whilst not interfering with or interrupting the interaction or potential for this between parent and child. The importance of not creating further disruption to the parent–child relationship needs to be taken seriously for the following reasons:

- The parent and child, although in difficulty, are still in the process of getting to know one another.
- The relationship between the two is shown in child development research to have a major underpinning role in advancing a child's cognitive, social and language development.
- At this stage, parents and children are spending probably the longest periods of time together (even if one or both parents go out to work), thereby having a particular opportunity for reparation to their relationship.

For the child, the normal developmental task in the second year is to use the parent as a 'secure base' (see Ch. 5). In infancy the attachment to the parent is the foundation for this, and from the second year the child will be using the internalised experience of this, plus the ongoing relationship with the parent to work out its own position in relation to the parent and the expanding world.

In the clinical population there has often been a disruption to the attachment between parent and infant and/or a later distortion of the 'secure base' phenomenon (Lieberman & Pawl 1990). There appear to be some points at which parents, after reflection in therapy, do pinpoint difficulties emerging with their child. The most common are at birth, at weaning, at the time the child becomes mobile and the child beginning playgroup or nursery. All these major adaptations have a common underlying process integral to the relationship, which is of a shift to greater separation and a need for a reorganisation of the patterns of relating.

Taking a frequently quoted and researched point of separation, the 'Strange Situation' test (Ainsworth et al 1978), it is clear to see that the most crucial aspect of achieving separation, even if momentarily distressing, is the child's belief that it will be able to regain contact with the primary attachment figure and that this contact brings reassurance and comfort/confidence. As Bowlby (1988) stated, a child can move away from the parent more easily only if the parent remains available for the child to return to when their explorations become too anxiety provoking (see Ch. 5).

Therefore, in considering the existing disruption in the relating of parent and child, the therapist needs to be aware that the child may turn to them as an emotionally available and thinking adult/parental figure. This may unwittingly reinforce the child's already internalised view that their parent is not reliable, and that they must look elsewhere. Many very young children, especially with 'avoidant' or 'disorganised' attachment classifications, show no hesitation in approaching the therapist for interaction, proximity, comfort or help, and pay little or no attention to their parent. There can undoubtedly be a pull within the therapist to respond generously to these overtures. This is especially so if the parent is constantly missing opportunities to look at and interact with their own child and are involved in describing a catalogue of negative behaviours or problems in the child. At times the conflict of interests between parent needs and child needs is hard for the therapist to manage.

It is possible to strike a balance of acknowledging the child, their feeling or view, but to turn and give this to the parent for thought and possible action. If the child makes a direct request, non-verbal or verbal to the therapist, the child's need is acknowledged but the therapist can then use this as an opportunity for the parent to respond. Although there is the risk that, in handing over the possible interaction to the parent, he or she will not respond, it also has many advantages that underpin the therapeutic alliance with the parent. These are:

- The parental aspect of the mother or father is tapped into, with the message from the therapist, that they have the capacity to make a helpful response to their child.
- It is more important that the infant or child turns to the parent for assistance and/or emotional care than to a relative stranger (i.e. the therapist). In promoting the child to access the parent appropriately, the child in turn can make a more direct appeal to the parent and this, with the therapist's confidence, can activate a belief in the parent that their child really does need them.
- The parent conversely does not see the therapist as the competent 'mummy' or 'daddy' that they feel themselves not to be. Many parents describe feeling undermined and deskilled in comparison to other adults' interaction with their child.

Situations where the therapist may need to have a more direct interpersonal relationship with child

If direct work is occurring with young children, either in an individual context, assessment, treatment or in a group, the above points need as much consideration but will be relevant in somewhat different contexts, for example in meeting the child and parent(s) before sessions, on reunion between parent and child. Additionally there may need to be a more graduated response in communicating with the child once the parent is present, but simultaneously introducing the idea that the child moves closer to the parent once more. Indications and contraindications for one-to-one therapy for young children will be discussed later.

PRESENTATION OF 'PROBLEMS' AND DIFFERENT APPROACHES TO ASSESSMENT

As with other age groups of children there are recurring similarities and clusters of particular problems or symptoms identified by referrers and presented to the CAMHS for assessment and/or treatment of young children aged 0–5 years. Specific to this age band, difficulties are framed often by a referring agency in terms of one or more of the following groups:

1. Difficulties of the infant or child in participating in or mastering activities of daily life, linked mainly to the routine tasks that have both a physical and a psychological component, such as feeding (before or after weaning), sleeping and toileting (before or after toilet training).
2. The child's behaviour – most often describing overt, active behaviours such as temper tantrums, aggression, opposition and overactivity, and less commonly identifying children whose behaviour is unusually subdued for this stage of life, perhaps withdrawn, mute or still.
3. Failure to achieve developmental milestones. This is often described by referrers in conjunction with one or both of the other main groups. Common areas of concern include the child not acquiring language (lack of pre-language skills infrequently identified), inability to socialise appropriately with peers, difficulty in learning, concentrating and playing.

In some referrals there may be a contextual picture of the child's family or social situation such as poor housing, overcrowding, marital conflict or separation, past or current child protection issues, parental ill-health. There may also be insights of the parent(s) included but experience has suggested that, whilst the information received in referrals is important, it is predominantly the adult's view of the 'problems' and the children's experience or perspective of these is lacking if not absent. One explanation for this is that many young children, even if they have acquired language, would find it hard to put their view of things into words. Therefore the assessment we carry out needs to find ways of creatively filling in a number of gaps, including the child's perspective and their experience of the difficulties, but also an exploration of how these appear in the most immediate environmental context for the child, that is within their relationship with their parent(s).

If we take the parent–child interaction and relationship as a central point, within and from which we can explore the variety of factors contributing to the presentation of problems in the child, we can also use this as a framework in terms of approaching the assessment in different ways.

The kind of influencing factors that each individual brings to the interaction with one another are represented diagrammatically in Figure 9.1. Initially mother and father are included in diagrams, and thereafter one parent will be used to illustrate different assessment frameworks. Figure 9.1 is an attempt to show many significant influences on parents and child but is by no means exhaustive, or suggestive that all these factors have clinical significance in every case.

How do we use the interaction between child and parent(s) to understand the extent to which behaviour, overt or absent, or lack of developmental progress in certain areas is attributable, and to what degree, to the parent–child relationship and how much they are linked to an intrinsic/genetic part of the child? (Boris et al 1997). This is a difficult and ambitious task and in many ways beyond our capacity. We rarely have the opportunity to work with the parent and infant from the beginning of life to see how the dyadic influences become established in certain patterns of interaction and behaviour. However, we do know that the care-giving environment directly affects brain development (Schore 1997) (see Ch. 5).

Take an example of a clinical presentation of a $1\frac{1}{2}$ year-old child who has a history of difficulty in feeding, of having frequent bouts of vomiting during milk and later solid feeds, and who now refuses largely to take any solid food even when completely mashed. She does not like to touch food, never wishes to hold a spoon and cannot tolerate any spills or messiness even when fed by her parents. She still regularly vomits during solid food meals.

We could understand this in terms of this child having a medical problem: reflux. Through repeatedly experiencing very unpleasant and

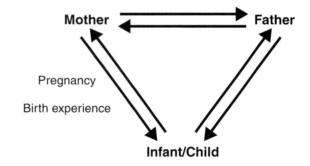

Childhood relationships with own parents

Current and past marital relationships

Mental and physical health

Truama/loss

Education

Employment

Gender of the child

Current family support

Mother ⟷ **Father**

Pregnancy

Birth experience

Infant/Child

Intrauterine experience

Birth and perinantal period

Gender

Temperament

Specific vulnerabilities

History of relationship with mother/father

Figure 9.1 Factors and influences brought by parents and their child to their relationship with one another.

distressing events at feed-times, she has now developed an anxious and avoidant response to solid food. Her continued vomiting could be considered a conditioned response to food passing down her throat. In addition, her parents have also been highly distressed by their daughter's feeding difficulties and now, as meal-times approach, feel increasing anxiety themselves.

On the other hand we could observe the current relationship between parent and child and hear some of its history. This gives a picture of the emotional states of those concerned, past and present. The mother presents as an extremely tense person, as if on the alert for danger. She says she cannot be still, has no patience if things do not go smoothly and stops feeding the child immediately anything disrupts the process, for instance when the child turns her head away from the spoon. Observation of the present interaction showed broadly two types of contact:

1. The girl's few attempts at play, her lack of contact with her mother for long periods, the mother's silence, rarely looking at her until a toy might fall, upon which she sharply says 'No! Bad girl'.
2. The other contrasting interaction was when she lay curled up on her mother's lap with a bottle of milk, and the mother then spoke warmly to her and stroked her hair.

Father, in the main, had no particular role or interaction with his daughter; he appeared to be on the periphery as an observer.

From this we could come to the conclusion that this child has probably experienced a lack of emotional availability from her mother and father in response to her developing need for greater autonomy. She has in addition received much anxiety and negativism from her mother which has been 'difficult to swallow' and subsequently has rejected what the mother has offered by way of food.

However, we cannot be sure that this is only a psychosomatic manifestation of emotional difficulties. By observing very real deficits in how parents and child relate to one another we cannot rule out that these may be present as contributing factors and need to think about both

presentations having relevance to the situation occurring now in the 'clinic' (clinic = health centre, outpatient service). Keeping a balance between both viewpoints is probably the most complex, but most realistic, way of understanding the interrelating influences that has made the feeding process such a painful experience for both the child and her parents. It has caused them to miss out shared activity time that can bring so much satisfaction, play and positive contact.

Where to begin in assessing a young child's difficulties

As a family is collected from the waiting room, a first impression is gained of how parent and child are together in an unfamiliar setting at a time of heightened stress. Useful observations to be made include:

1. The proximity the child keeps to the parent.
2. Joint activity between child or parent or whether the child is playing alone.
3. Parent's communication to the child about leaving the waiting room or not.
4. Parent's ability to help the child to make the transition from the waiting room into the clinic room.

Examples of common presentations:

• The child is on the move frequently, facing away from the parent. There is no communication, although the child may try to engage a stranger also sitting in the area in a non-verbal interaction or conversation. The parent sits looking away from the child, silently. On our introduction and greeting, the parent will often respond to the therapist and call briefly to the child, perhaps just using their name. Children often do one of two things: abandon toys and rush to parent's side or make no evident response. Parent–child conflict with the latter can lead to a threat to leave the child or engagement with the child but in an angry fashion.

• The child sits with the parent, or stands nearby; both are engaged in looking at a book or toy. The child retains proximity as the parent greets the therapist, and begins to move. Some

Equally, parenting couples may become aware of there being some exclusive difficulties between themselves that are impinging on their capacity to think about and interact with the children. Depending on the experience of the therapist and other available resources, couple work can be interchanged with parent–child work, or a couple may be referred on so that this work runs in parallel.

Individual work with young children

Embarking on individual work with such young children needs careful thought. If this idea does come to mind then, before acting, it would be worth taking a moment to consider on what thoughts and feelings, particularly the therapist's, it is based. This point is raised because, when relationships between parents and young children have become disturbed, conflictual and distressing, there is often a heightened intensity of emotion and worry around that can easily be taken on board by the therapist. In some cases there may be an unconscious wish on the parents' part metaphorically to 'hand over' the child to the therapist, because of anger and projection on to the child and/or their own destroyed confidence in their role as parent. However, this period of time in a parent and child's life together is also perhaps the most optimal time to redress gaps, failures and conflicts as it is a time of rapid development. For these reasons, work with the parent and child together is often indicated on a trial basis in the first instance.

Some indications for individual work with 3–5 year olds include:

• A young child established in a long-term foster placement or with adopted parents who has, in previous attachment relationships, experienced trauma, neglect or abuse. Parallel parent–child work may be important with a different worker in order to facilitate the child's current attachment and relationship.

• Where the primary care-giver is experiencing acute difficulties such as physical illness requiring hospitalisation or severe mental health problems. Again, the length of time for which individual work is planned should be determined by the primary goal, that the parent

(if this is possible) take up fully the responsibility for the child's emotional well-being again, which may be facilitated by some parent work or parent–child work running in parallel.

• Where the relationship has broken down to such a degree that the child has become extremely defensive to the approach of the parent and where conflict is frequent and volatile. This is found in few instances, even working in a population with a high incidence of social deprivation and severe intergenerational parenting difficulties.

CONCLUSION

The work described in this chapter draws on the clinical practice developed in an under-fives service over a number of years, which has combined infant/child development research with attachment and psychoanalytical theories. It has aimed to provide an understanding of the interpersonal context in which the difficulties of young children arise. This context is known from recent research and from clinical experience to have particular significance in the early years of a child's life. An attempt has been made to describe different levels at which a child and family's problems can be investigated and then worked on in treatment. For the purposes of introducing such a framework, approaches have been described as separate entities, but it is hoped that the relationship between them will be considered further by practitioners and stimulate a flexible way of thinking about and offering help to parents and young children.

ACKNOWLEDGEMENTS

The parent–child work described in this chapter has been developed jointly by the author and B. Kiely, Sister in Child Mental Health. The author also thanks Dr Maureen Marks for her comments.

REFERENCES

Ainsworth, M D S, Blehar M C, Waters E, Wall S 1978 Patterns of attachment: a psychological study of the strange situation. Erlbaum, Hillsdale, NJ

Boris N W, Fueyo M, Zeanah C H 1997 The clinical assessment of attachment in children under five. Journal of the American Academy of Child and Adolescent Psychiatry 36(2):291–293

Bowlby J 1988 A secure base. Clinical applications of attachment theory. Routledge, London

Brazelton T B, Koslowski B, Main M 1974 The origins of reciprocity: the early mother–infant interaction. In: Lewis M, Rosenblum L (eds) The effect of the infant on its caregiver. Wiley, Chichester, UK

Brazelton T B, Cramer B G 1991 The earliest relationship: parents, infants and the drama of early attachment. Karnac Books, London

Fraiberg S 1982 Pathological defenses in infancy. Psychoanalytic Quarterly L1:612–635

Fraiberg S (ed) 1989 Assessment and therapy of disturbances in infancy. Jason Aronson, Northvale, New Jersey

Lieberman A F, Pawl J H 1990 Disorders of attachment and secure base behaviour in the second year of life. In: Greenberg M T, Cicchetti D, Cummings E M (eds) Attachment in the preschool years. University of Chicago Press, Chicago

Murray L, Cooper P J (eds) 1977 Postpartum depression and child development. Guilford Press, New York

Piontelli A 1992 From fetus to child: an observational and psychoanalytic study. Routledge, London

Schore A N 1997 Interdisciplinary developmental research as a source of clinical models. In: Moskowitz M, Monk C, Kaye C, Ellman S J (eds) The neurobiological and developmental basis for psychotherapeutic intervention. Jason Aronson, Northvale, New Jersey

Stern D 1977 The first relationship. Harvard University Press, Cambridge, Massachusetts

Stern D 1985 The interpersonal world of the infant. Basic Books, New York

Trevarthen C 1980 Foundations of intersubjectivity: development of interpersonal and co-operative understanding in infants. In: Olson D (ed) The social foundations of language and thought. W W Norton, New York

Tronick E Z 1989 Emotions and emotional communication in infants. American Psychologist February:112–119

Tronick E Z, Weinberg M K 1997 Depressed mothers and infants: failure to form dyadic states of conciousness. In: Murray L, Cooper P J (eds) Postpartum depression and child development. Guilford Press, New York, p 54

Winnicott D W 1992 Anxiety associated with insecurity. In: Through paediatrics to psychoanalysis. Karnac Books, London

Winnicott D W 1986 Babies and their mothers. Addison-Wesley, Reading, Massachusetts

FURTHER READING

Brazelton T B 1992 Touchpoints. Your child's emotional and behavioural development. Viking, London

Osborne E (series ed) 1992 Understanding your baby/1 year old/2 year old/etc. Rosendale Press, London

Putnam F W 1997 Dissociation in children and adolescents. A developmental perspective. Guilford, New York

Raphael-Leff J 1991 Psychological processes of childbearing. Chapman & Hall, London

Weininger O 1993 View from the cradle. Children's emotions in everyday life. Karnac Books, London

Winnicott D W 1993 Talking to parents. Addison-Wesley, Harlow tunities (Florey & Greene 1997, Reid & Kolvin 1993). Problems in peer relationships can be addressed directly as difficult feelings and problematic situations arise, with the presence of other children providing different avenues for learning and change. Children can serve as role models for interactions and dealing with problems, and there is a chance to try out new ways of relating in a safe environment. Groups may also be therapeutic in their potential to offer an experience of belonging and seeing that others too have problems. Children can share their experiences and offer support and objective feedback, often in a way that their peers are willing to accept.

Whether the particular group being offered is therapeutic for a specific child depends on several considerations. Age is one, in that groups for primary school children tend to be most cohesive when they have no more than a 3-year age band. How similar or different a child is in comparison to other members is another. When the focus is on developing peer relationships, being with a mixture of personalities allows for flexibility of role models and a range of interactive experiences. Alternatively, for children suffering from traumatic experiences, for example bereavement or sexual abuse, being with others who have had similar experiences may be therapeutically advantageous. Difference in gender or other factors can set a single member apart from the group, and it is useful to avoid this if possible.

Family work

Relationship problems within the family, or shared experiences that the family wish to address, are probably best addressed with some form of family work. Parent–child approaches discussed in Chapter 9 will be relevant, although children of school age will have more capacity to communicate their views, reason and negotiate. Approaches discussed in Chapter 7 will also be suitable.

Individual work

Many problems can be addressed in individual work (see Ch. 6), but it is particularly useful when a child is attempting to make sense of traumatic life experiences, learning to trust, or developing or integrating inner resources. It may enable some children to engage in group work or participate more successfully in family work.

SOME THERAPEUTIC CONSIDERATIONS

Working together

When offering treatment for children of this age it is usually important to think not only about the working relationship with the child, but also that with the parent, the school and any other professionals involved with the child and family. Whether or not a child's therapy begins and continues really comes down to the parent, and thus it is crucial that they are considered throughout the process, whatever the level of their involvement may be. At the very least, there will be a need for liaison, but they may also be involved in home programmes or more directly in parallel treatment such as parent or family work. Communication with schools or other professionals, such as social workers or other therapists, will also be important to ensure that everyone is working towards the same goals.

Meetings

An initial meeting to discuss why treatment is being offered, what it will entail and the expectations of all involved can encourage everyone in working together from the very beginning. The inclusion of children gives them the opportunity to see that the problems they are having can be talked about and tackled. It also gives the chance to minimise any anxieties about why it is that they are going to be coming to a clinic. Many children view themselves as 'bad' or 'naughty' and expect to be punished or sent away, so they may be very worried about what this 'therapy' is all about. Hearing more about what will be happening may be a relief. When a parent is not going to be included in the therapy, for example when individual or group work is being offered, it may be important for the child to see that the parent gives permission and is supportive of the process. This may help the child to view therapy as something helpful, as well as allow them to accept something for themselves, separately from their parent.

Defining what it is that is being worked toward and clarifying who will be doing what can be very helpful in encouraging all those involved to see therapy as a shared responsibility that includes the child, parents and occupational therapist, and possibly others. Written contracts with clear goals and tasks for all involved, can be useful (see Box 10.4). They can then serve as a reference when reviewing progress and refining goals. Practicalities such as dates of attendance, breaks, punctuality, cancellations, relevant policies and procedures can be discussed at this time and included in a contract, or provided as a handout. If parental consent is required for any procedures, for example use of video, it is important to obtain this in writing.

Regular review meetings are useful so that everyone involved has the opportunity to receive feedback as well as air their views, ask questions or raise concerns. Goals and plans can then be revised as necessary.

Liaising with parents

If a child is being seen individually or in a group, liaison may also take place on a relatively informal basis when children are dropped off or collected or in 'emergency meetings' when there has been a serious incident or worries have arisen about a child's safety and protection.

It is common for parents to feel some anxiety about getting feedback on their child, especially as many will have been experiencing problems with their child for some time. Some may expect complaints about their child or criticisms of their parenting, while others may worry that something harmful will have happened to their child while they have been apart. These anxieties can be exacerbated if feedback is to take place in front of other parents or children, as sometimes happens when children attend a group, and parents may react by arriving late or sending someone else to collect their child. Feedback in such situations can be limited to that which is supportive and encouraging to parents, and potentially more threatening issues kept for private meetings.

Sometimes other forms of communication may be useful, especially if time is limited. Written feedback in the form of 'link books', which outline the focus of a session, the child's achievements and allow for parents to write their comments, may offer an alternative. Colouring charts, stamps or stickers, with or without written feedback, are a popular alternative for younger children (see Fig. 10.1).

Home programmes

Parents may be encouraged to support their child's treatment by setting up opportunities or a suitable environment, or actually doing activities with their child at home. Some examples include establishing a quiet work corner, assisting in arrangements for inviting another child over to play after school, or setting aside 20 minutes a day for a programme of specified activities. A realistic assessment of the family's resources, the parent's

---

Box 10.4 Example of a contract for a 10-year-old child

1. Luke is going to attend the After School Group every Thursday afternoon from 4–6 pm, beginning on September 24th.
2. Luke is working on the following goals:
   a) To be able to wait his turn.
   b) To be able to sort out arguments without hurting anybody.
3. Mrs S will help Luke with any homework from the group.
4. Ms P and Ms B, Luke's class teacher, will meet at least once this term.
5. A review meeting will be held on December 10th with Luke, Mrs S, Ms B and Ms P.
Signed:

. . . .

. . . .

. . . .

. . . .

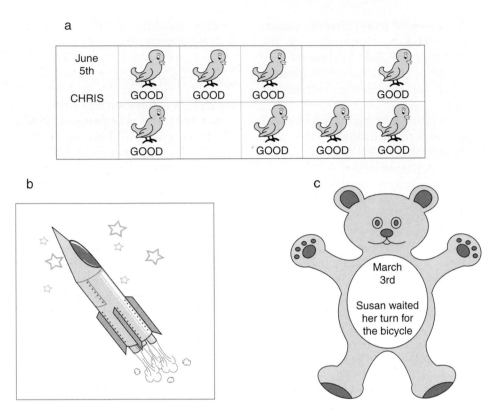

Figure 10.1 Examples of visual feedback for younger children. (a) Stamps indicating whether or not a child has succeeded in following the two rules of staying in place (top row) and being friendly to others (bottom row) in each activity. (b) Colouring chart, where the child colours in a star for each time he or she shared. (c) Sticker (using double-sided tape) with feedback for parent on the child's social efforts. See Appendix for supplier of manufactured stampers, stickers and certificates.

understanding of what it is they are being asked to do, and the parent–child relationship will influence the effectiveness of such an approach.

Parallel work with parents

Sometimes it is possible to offer parents sessions either individually or in a group, which provide support and the opportunity to explore any difficulties they may have in assisting their child. Alternatively, other members of the team may offer this work in parallel. Provided there is good communication between the professionals, issues can be addressed from both the child's and the parent's perspective. For example, if listening is a topic in a group for 9–11-year-olds, then in a parallel parent group, or an individual parent ses-

sion, the issue of how parents listen to their children may be explored. This way of working does, however, require a considerable amount of time, given the necessary planning and liaison.

Liaising with schools

Information may be shared with regard to specific concerns and progress, and link books can be used between school, home and clinic. Many children of this age require additional support in school and the occupational therapist may be involved in the assessment procedure of their special educational needs. Clarification of roles may be necessary if a paediatric occupational therapist is also involved, for example if a child has a physical disability.

Security

Ensuring that the therapeutic environment is a place where children can feel emotionally as well as physically safe is important regardless of whether individual, group or family work is being offered. If children are overwhelmed by anxiety or preoccupied with having to protect themselves, they are unlikely to have much energy left to learn from their experiences and from what others have to offer.

There are different ingredients that go into creating a secure environment, but two essential ones are a supportive and understanding attitude, and a capacity to set limits. This is not unlike the way in which parents facilitate their child's well-being and development.

Conveying an interest in understanding what a child is experiencing or what it is like 'to be in their shoes' can be very containing. An individual child may benefit in terms of feeling understood and then be more able to think about the situation they are in, possibly finding a solution. If there are other children present, they may have the opportunity to learn how others can be treated with tolerance and understanding, and to be more open about themselves (see Box 10.5).

Box 10.5 Case example : Ivan

Ivan, aged 6, said that he had got an injection in his arm and that it hurt. Harry, aged 5, called out that Ivan was a baby, and that he, Harry, never cried. The therapist commented that injections could be frightening and that it it might be hard not to cry. Harry sat quietly for a moment, then said that he was scared because his dad was in prison and he didn't know whether he would ever come out.

As many of the children who are offered treatment have little trust in themselves or others, it can be helpful and containing to have clear expectations from the beginning about what is acceptable and what is not. In individual work, this might be as simple as talking with a child about staying in the room and about it not being 'OK' to hurt anybody. In group work, it may be important to have additional expectations about behaviour in the group and how the group will function in addressing problems, especially around the issue of how other children are treated. This can create more of a sense of predictability in the group.

Rules can be particularly valuable, especially for children who may need to develop their self-control and ability to get on with others. When framed in a positive manner (e.g. 'We stay in our places') rather than negative commands (e.g. 'No leaving the room'), they can provide guidelines for behaviour which can then be easily encouraged amongst the children. For the youngest of this age range, usually one or two rules is all that they can remember, even when reviewed regularly, whereas older children may manage up to four. Children are usually concerned with fairness and can be encouraged to take some responsibility for monitoring the rules and discussing when they are broken. Older children may also be involved in setting some of the rules.

The balance that is struck between supporting or understanding and setting limits will depend on many factors. In individual work, children's different needs can be considered. For example, a very chaotic and overactive child may require firm limits before being able to settle to anything or listen. Another child may continually test limits and boundaries, particularly at the beginning of treatment, and may need a very consistent response over and over again in order to feel safe. As treatment progresses, both may be encouraged to make more choices about their behaviour and to develop their own self-control. Alternatively, a self-conscious and anxious child may benefit from permission to explore gradually beyond their strict controls and to see that there are not such disastrous consequences as might have been imagined. In groups, individual as well as group needs must be considered, and more limits may need to be set as out-of-control behaviour can quickly escalate and spread amongst group members, especially if leaders appear uncertain about managing the situation (Woods 1993). An overly controlled group, however, can inhibit growth and make it less likely that what is learned will be generalised to other aspects of the child's life.

Predictable routines, such as regular sessions set at the same time and day each week and the use of activity timetables for groups, may also promote a sense of security. The pleasure of being able to anticipate what will be happening next is often very obvious in the children who come for treatment, as is the anxiety that can be evoked by sudden changes. Where possible, it is important to allow children time to prepare for known changes, such as holidays, endings, and children or leaders joining or leaving a group. Talking about these events as well as unexpected changes, such as absences, makes it less likely that the children will express their uncertainty and distress through actions.

Rituals can bring children together as well as help them to feel more able to face change. Strength seems to come from knowing what will be happening and feeling that there are others – present, past and future – who will experience something of the same. Take, for example, a group of 5–7-year-olds who met regularly at a day programme. A ritual was established for saying goodbye whenever a member left. They knew that each of them would have a turn to hold a cardboard model of a present and tell the child leaving about one thing they would like to give them as a leaving present. Often, a lot of thought would go into this with children saying things like: 'I would buy you a train set. You always liked playing with it here.' or 'I'd give you a dog to play with so you won't miss us too much. I'll miss you.' They always chose to participate, even if they needed a little help, for example having another child say it with them.

Communication

The way in which children communicate often means an adjustment on the part of the occupational therapist, both in terms of understanding what a child is saying and in conveying information to a child. This may be a simple consequence of the maturity of the child or it may be that a child has specific difficulties in communicating or in relating to present additional challenges.

There is often a dramatic difference in the way in which children of infant school age communicate, compared with those of junior school age. The younger children tend to be less skilled verbally and may present with limited vocabulary, poor pronunciation and difficulties in organising their language output. They may not always converse logically and they may move between reality and fantasy. They may make specific references to their life experiences, but without providing the necessary information in order for others to know what they are talking about. For instance, they may refer to someone they know, events in a television programme or a place they have been, and expect others to know all about it. These difficulties usually are less pronounced in the upper end of this age range, but many still have difficulties in conveying what is on their mind or what they are feeling.

Making sense of child's communications can take a fair amount of effort on the part of the occupational therapist and it is often necessary to attend to the verbal content as well as what the child may be conveying non-verbally or through their play. In addition to gaining a better understanding of the child, such efforts show the child that they are an interesting person to be listened to. The occupational therapist's comments may also indicate that there are words to express feelings and thoughts. It is important, however, that children take an active part in learning to express themselves in ways that can be understood. Thus, a child may need encouragement to slow down, to provide more details, or to make a distinction between whether it really happened or whether it was a wish.

Many of the children who come for treatment are not very receptive to the communications of others. They may not be very trusting or they may have significant difficulties in self-control and easily become overly excited, anxious, upset or disorganised. Building a relationship is the first step in motivating children to listen to instructions, guidance, information and commands that the occupational therapist may wish to deliver. In order to focus and take in what is said to them, however, they may need others to alter the way in which information is provided. A hushed voice and a slower speed, for instance, may help a child who is over-excited to calm to a level where more information can be received. Similarly, for children who have been traumatised and are likely to be sensitised to threat (Perry et al 1995), non-confrontative directions may be more effective in terms of gaining the child's attention and cooperation than commands. Others may benefit from additional visual cues, such as placing a finger to one's mouth or other gestures, and a simplification of language.

Although, for the most part, communication is likely to take place in the context of play or other activities, the occupational therapist may work with other professionals to provide activities that focus primarily on verbal communication. 'Group meetings' or 'circle time', for instance, may provide an opportunity for children to express themselves verbally and to practise their listening and turn-taking skills.

Children may also learn about communication through observation and, when there are two therapists working with a group or family, there are additional interactions and communications. Even when disagreements arise, which is bound to happen, there are valuable opportunities to see that differences can be addressed and resolved through communication, either in deciding to discuss them later, taking a few minutes aside to talk, or in negotiating a solution within the therapy.

Playing and working

The belief that there is therapeutic value in 'doing' has long been held by the occupational therapy profession (Rebeiro 1998). It is considered that through 'doing' there is the opportunity to develop skills and capacities, to get to know the self and the environment, physical and social, and to experience pleasure and a sense of competence.

For children of school age, purposeful and meaningful 'doing' in everyday life can be said to consist increasingly of working as well as playing. Academic learning, taking lessons, for example in music or swimming, being a member of a sports team or a club, and engaging in hobbies such as model-making, all require some degree of working. That is, there are external restrictions on what children can do and how they do it, and the process may not necessarily be enjoyable in itself, but persistence may result in eventual gains such as achievement or social acceptance. This is in contrast to playing, in which children are more or less in charge of what they do, where the pleasure comes primarily from the process itself, and there is the freedom to suspend reality (Bundy 1997, Canadian Association of Occupational Therapists 1996).

Promoting children's capacity for playing or for working may be aims of the therapeutic intervention, but, equally, facilitating children's active engagement in playing and working may be used as a means of attaining other goals in treatment, such as exploring and mastering troubling experiences, developing specific skills or improving relationships.

Depending on the needs that individual children present at any particular moment, the occupational therapist may take a more active role in facilitating either playing or working, although these two processes may not be so distinct in practice. If, for example, children are being encouraged to learn about their own power (West 1992), to express or discover themselves (Winnicott 1971), to work out a creative way forward with regard to a problem (Smith & Simon 1984), or to relax and have a little light-hearted fun, then playing may provide more of a learning experience. Working, on the other hand, may offer opportunities for dealing with the frustration of having limits imposed by others or the environment, and learning about the benefits of self-discipline and control.

Playing and having fun together can help children to establish or rebuild connections with others, but a degree of external structure may help children to feel more comfortable and safe when they do not know others very well or are unsure about what will happen. Games with rules or making things alongside one another may be more tolerable in the early stages of a group, or for some children beginning therapy.

There are different ways in which the occupational therapist can facilitate children's active engagement in doing. One is through provision of an appropriate environment. There are some children who have a well-developed capacity to play and respond to the provision of suitable toys and materials, but many need to experience the light-hearted attitude, flexibility and playful responsiveness of another in order to get going. Similarly, some children may be able to apply themselves to the task of working, while others benefit from clear choices, reminders of the goal being worked towards, breaking down of the task into manageable steps, and another's expectation that there is a time for work.

Ensuring that the challenges are kept to a manageable level, either through structuring of the activity, adaptations or the support that is provided, will also facilitate children's playing or working. Challenges that are at too high a level may be overwhelming, and some children may respond by engaging in less purposeful and meaningful behaviour, such as repetitive actions, controlling of others or distracting conversations, while others may react aggressively or collapse in helplessness. Such behaviours can have a negative impact on children's sense of competency as well as their relationships with others. Challenges that are too low, however, not only lead to boredom, but deprive children of those moments that allow them to experience the full potential of their resources and of the opportunities that they need to grow and develop.

Playing requires that children express an aspect of self, either through initiation of an idea or through action. This involves a degree of risk and some children benefit from extra space, for example through providing extra time to respond or giving choice, and minimization of pressure or expectations. On the other hand, in working, children need to be able to delay self-gratification and tolerate the difficult feelings that may be evoked in waiting or considering others. Thus, noting when children do exert such efforts can encourage their development in this area. For example, commenting on how angry a child feels when another child is not playing fairly, and on the effort needed for self-control so that he does not hurt anyone, can encourage the child to tolerate such difficult feelings and to be aware of their capacity for self-control.

Motivation

Children are usually easily motivated to engage in therapeutic activities, playing or working, provided that these are within their capabilities and are age appropriate in terms of interest. Sometimes, however, more novelty, the inclusion of a favourite theme or character, an idea about what they will be doing with their finished product, or other adaptations are necessary to make an activity more attractive. Using intrinsic sources of motivation such as these can encourage children to take pleasure in doing and develop their competence in task-related skills and capacities.

There are times, however, when more extrinsic sources of motivation are worth consideration. For instance, a child who is needing to persist at practising a skill in order to achieve a goal, or children having to learn new ways of behaving or interacting with others, may benefit from the extra incentive of external rewards.

Adult attention can be very effective, especially with the younger of this age range. Praise that is consistent, immediate and contingent for specific behaviours can be very effective in helping children to alter their behaviour. For example, an impulsive child may be praised each time they remember to wait in turn, while a very shy and anxious child may receive praise whenever a reply is made to others' questions, even if to say, 'I don't know'. Such reinforcement may help children to persist in their efforts until there comes a time when they begin to experience the benefits inherent in behaving in these new ways. For example, a child who shares for the first time may not necessarily receive positive feedback from peers, or perceive their receptiveness. However, receiving praise for effort may motivate the child to try again, increasing the likelihood of eventually experiencing a more positive response from others.

For some children tangible rewards, such as stickers, certificates, edible treats or small toys, may be more effective sources of motivation. Children who do not have much trust in what adults say, or those who do not take in verbal praise very easily, perhaps due to poor attention or listening skills, may be more responsive to visual reinforcement. Such possibilities may have been the case when a reward system was implemented for a 6-year-old boy with significant behavioural problems who had not been responding to adult encouragement and praise. Upon receiving a sticker for the first time, he beamed and then announced: 'I've never been good before!'. The relative permanency of some tangible rewards may also be beneficial in that the children can show them to their parents or other significant people and receive additional recognition for their efforts. It is important, however, to plan for a gradual decrease in the use of rewards, so that children are eventually encouraged to rely more on their own experiences of being effective in their physical and social environments.

Other behavioural methods such as sanctions (e.g. 'There will be no biscuit if you continue kicking') or time out may be appropriate in some cases, but are most effective when their use is infrequent and the therapist's emphasis is on noticing the positives. Experiences of deprivation, rejection, loss or excessive punitive discipline tend to make it less likely for children to believe that there will be anything good or pleasurable anyway, so that having something taken away or being removed usually does not work as an incentive for them to try harder. Instead, it can increase feelings of anger and despondency that anything can be different.

The need to belong to a group and be accepted by peers is another important source of motivation for children of this age. Rewards that work in individual therapy or at home may not be so effective in a group if they mean that a child is singled out from peers. For example, a 6-year-old boy may respond enthusiastically to a chart with a moveable batman figure that 'flies' up a building when he cooperates at home with the morning routine. The same chart in a group, however, may well be rejected.

Children may participate in activities that they might otherwise be reluctant to try, in order to be part of the group. Similarly, they may try to follow the example of other children who have managed to make changes. In well-established open groups, it is common for children who have been in the group for some time to take pleasure in encouraging newer members. For example, a child may comment: 'I used to get into loads of fights when I first came here, but I'm getting better at sorting them out without beating someone up'. Confrontation from peers in the context of a supportive group can also motivate children to make changes. For example, a 10-year-old girl may be more likely to accept that she sometimes encourages the other children to get angry with her by her provocative behaviour if she is told this by the other children rather than by the occupational therapist. With encouragement, they are also likely to be able to offer some insights into why she behaves this way and to encourage her to behave in other ways that will lead to friendships rather than always being the odd one out.

Safety and protection

Children of school age are still relatively dependent and thus, when working with children separately from their parents, it is the occupational therapist's responsibility to ensure their care, protection and safety. When a child is ill, gets injured or makes a disclosure in treatment, the occupational therapist will need to be ready to respond. There are usually procedures to follow in each place of work and it is important to be up to date with these.

Children sometimes do present with dangerous behaviour in treatment and the occupational therapist must be prepared to deal with this situation should it arise. This is especially important to consider when running groups, where one child's dangerous behaviour may also threaten the safety of others, and may spark off other children's out-of-control and dangerous behaviour. There are some issues that can be considered before beginning work so that the potential for crises is minimised. The physical environment, for instance, needs to be appropriate for children who may at times act impulsively or lose control. For example, using a room that can be exited by only one door, the use of child locks on main exits, and restricted windows may be necessary to ensure that children do not run out of a room or building.

It is also important that those working with children feel able to provide a secure environment, as discussed above. Thus, with groups in particular, careful selection of referrals is recommended so that the composition and size is manageable. For example, a maximum of eight junior school children, some with significant behavioural problems, may be fine for two experienced therapists within a supportive organisation, while the number may be limited to four in the case of two therapists who are setting up groups for the first time.

Despite all efforts and best intentions to prevent dangerous or out-of-control behaviour, there are still likely to be times when such moments arise, especially in groups. One reason for this is that the therapist can never really know about all the events that may trigger a response in a child. What disturbs one child may pass unnoticed by others. For instance, a child who has been traumatised by abuse and the threat of being taken away by police may suddenly jump up in the middle of a group activity, shouting angrily and shaking a chair over their head, having heard the approaching sound of a siren. It is helpful for group leaders to decide on the ways in which they will respond to dangerous or out-of-control behaviour so that there is a plan to fall back on at such times. This may include a procedure in which a child sits with a parent instead of attending the therapy, or the use of holding or restraint as a last resort. Training is recommended for the latter option and it is prudent to have the backing of the organisation on this matter.

Time to reflect

Evaluation is an essential part of the occupational therapy process, and making time for it ensures that interventions are meeting a child's needs, that progress is monitored, and that there is time to prepare for changes or endings. Sometimes there is not adequate thinking time in the actual sessions with children, owing to the high levels of activity, and sometimes the feelings that are evoked in working with children can be unsettling to the therapist. Setting aside time to reflect is therefore important, both in understanding what has occurred in a session and in finding solutions to problems. For example, it is not uncommon for group leaders to find that tensions arise within their working relationship. Having time to think about their feelings and behaviour, for example competiveness or strongly opposed feelings, as well as the ways in which the children might play one leader off against the other or expect an inequality of power, may enable the therapists to understand what is happening and to find ways of working in a more united manner.

With groups, it is necessary to think about the group as a whole and the processes that occur between children, as well as the individuals within it. One child, for example, may stand out as particularly difficult in a group due to disruptive behaviour. It could be that the child is not well placed in a group, but it may also be that the child is acting unconsciously on the group's behalf, perhaps as a spokesperson expressing the anger for the group or as a scapegoat, becoming a receptable for the split-off and intolerable parts of others (Horwitz 1983). If there are group issues, such as upset about a change of group leader or insufficient space for individual expression, excluding the identified child for individual treatment would be an inappropriate solution for meeting individual and group needs, and could lead to another child taking up the empty role.

Just as it is important for the occupational therapist to take time to reflect, it is useful to think with children about what happens in a session. In the heat of the moment it may be that the occupational therapist needs to do most of the thinking, but gradually children may be prompted to do a little more thinking themselves. Thinking back over an incident or a session can encourage children to develop more of a capacity to reflect, to be more aware of choices, and to control actively their own behaviour.

THE ACTIVITIES

The choice of activity or combinations of activities is determined by treatment goals, but also by what is happening in the here and now. A considerable amount of flexibility with regard to planned activities and having extra ideas 'up one's sleeve' makes it more likely that individual or group needs will be met.

Adult-directed activities

Skill oriented. These activities are selected and structured by the occupational therapist in order to help children develop particular skills or aspects of their performance.

Social. Children with relationship difficulties may benefit from opportunities to learn and practise particular social skills. These may be simple in nature, such as greeting others or saying 'no', or more complex, such as joining a group of peers or responding to teasing. To capture children's interest in learning a particular skill, stories may be told through dramatisation and puppets, a video may be used so that children can watch themselves and their peers, or they may plan and create a book, play or video for younger children. Role-play can be used to practise a skill, although younger children need concrete reminders in order to keep to the purpose of the role-play. So, for example, if doing a role-play on joining other children in play, younger ones may be asked actually to play a particular game, such as snakes and ladders, to enable them to assume their roles, while older ones may be able to create an imaginary situation from their own experiences. Selected activities or games may provide the opportunity to practise particular skills, for example verbal communication or assertiveness, and they may be graded in terms of the challenge, for instance through an increase in the degree of competition. Activities that focus on the development of social skills can also form part of a more structured social skills training programme, involving instruction, modelling, rehearsal and feedback, as well as other techniques such as positive reinforcement and homework tasks (Cartledge & Milburn 1996).

Cognitive. Activites that focus on underlying beliefs, feelings or thinking and coping skills may be used as a means of helping children to develop more adaptive strategies for performing tasks or solving interpersonal problems. Young children who are overly anxious in their performance, for example, may be encouraged to interact with a teddy bear puppet who talks with them about everyone making mistakes. Older children who have difficulties with peers might play a game in which they generate solutions to problematic situations, for example being teased by a particular child in the playground. To make it more fun, cards with pictures depicting general solutions such as 'ignore', 'find someone to play with', 'tell an adult' (Camp & Bash 1981) might be awarded for each new and different idea. In helping children to identify their own feelings and those of others, a game might be played in which they take turns to spin a dial that can point to one of ten cartoon facial expressions. After identifying the feeling, the child tells of a time when they had that feeling. Such activities may be part of more formal training programmes, such as interpersonal problem-solving or cognitive restructuring programmes (Pellegrini 1994, Spence 1994).

Physical. Direct practice of skills can be presented in the form of enjoyable and meaningful activities. For example, a 9-year-old child with illegible handwriting may be encouraged to practise word spacing by writing secret messages, making the list of ingredients for cooking, or writing to a penfriend. Sensorimotor activities, such as those described by Fink (1989), may be used to help children develop their capacities for performing certain tasks, as may a programme of graded activities. For example, an 8-year-old wanting to learn to ride a bicycle may be encouraged to play balancing games on a large therapy ball and barrel, to cycle a stationary bicycle during games of I-spy and bean bag toss, and then graduate to riding a bicycle with stabilizers and finally practise on their own bicycle.

Task oriented. Structured activities that produce an end-product are useful for children who have difficulties in organising themselves and completing what they begin. They can be graded to allow a sense of achievement to be experienced and a well-presented end-product can offer concrete feedback with regard to their competence. They can also be used for practising and integrating other skills, whether these are social, cognitive or physical. In groups, interacting during task-oriented activities may be less threatening, but the physical and cognitive challenges do

Appendix:

Suppliers of standardised tests

NFER Nelson Publishing
Darville House
2 Oxford Road East
Windsor
SL4 1DF
UK
Tel: 01753 858961

Bruininks–Oseretsky Test of Motor Proficiency (Bruininks 1978)

The Psychological Corporation
32 Jamestown Road
London
NW1 7BY
Tel: 0207 4244200

Movement Assessment Battery for Children (Henderson & Sugden 1992)

Motor-Free Visual Perception Test (Colarusso & Hamill 1972)

Test of Visual Perceptual Skills (Gardner 1982)

Test of Visual Motor Skills (Gardner 1986)

Western Psychological Services
12031 Wilshire Boulevard
Los Angeles
California
USA

Sensory Integration and Praxis Tests (Ayres 1989)

Suppliers of stickers, stampers and certificates.

Super Stickers
PO Box 55
4 Balloo Avenue
Bangor
County Down
BT19 7PJ
UK

11

Occupational therapy with adolescents

Anna Flanigan

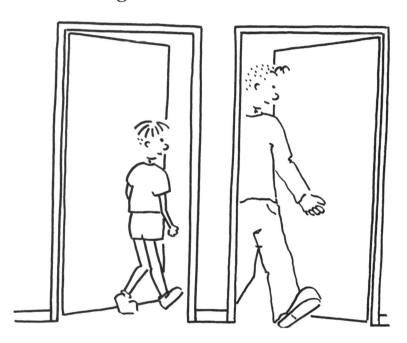

INTRODUCTION

Most people have powerful memories of their adolescence, whether pleasurable or painful. In his training paper 'An introduction to adolescence' Harold Marchant (1987) suggests an instructive exercise for those thinking of working with this age group whereby participants are asked to bring in an item that reminds them of, and conjures up, their own adolescence. Mine would be a jacket I bought in 1970 in Dorothy

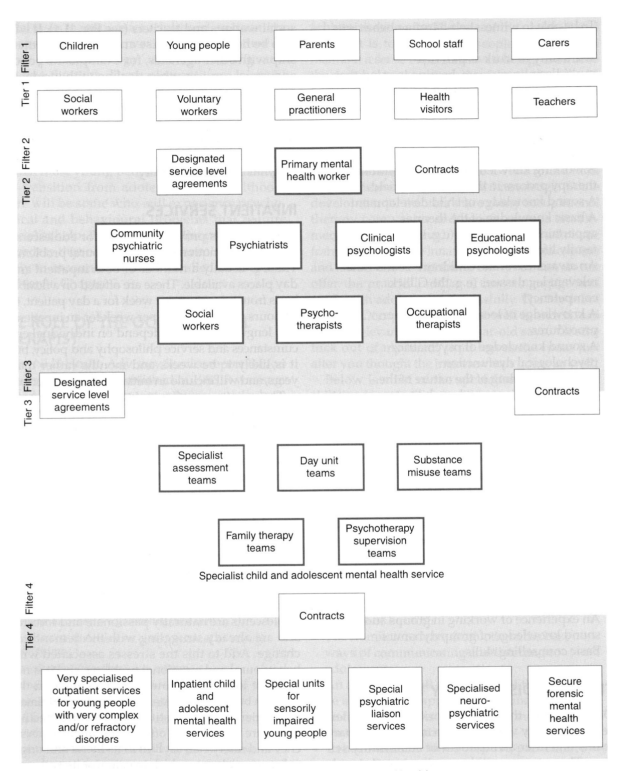

Figure 11.1   Organisation of service delivery in child and adolescent mental health.

worst, these units encourage dependency on an unreal, cloistered world from which it is hard to move on and away. This can be the case for both clients and staff. As a member of the team, the occupational therapist must find ways of coping with the day-to-day emotional challenge. The sources of support will be from within the team and from personal support structures. The issue of support and supervision is explored further in Chapter 14.

The role of the occupational therapist can help. Adolescents, on the whole, want to work in the here and now rather than the past. Their main developmental task is to cope successfully with the present in order to move into the future. The occupational therapist, by dealing with present and future roles and activities, encouraging self-reliance and promoting self-esteem, can keep a perspective on the real world and retain a balanced view of the work and the workplace.

THE COMMUNITY SETTING

In a community setting the role of the occupational therapist may be less well defined than in an inpatient unit. For example, some teams do not differentiate between professionals and may describe team members as child mental health professionals. The struggle between professional identity and team membership is ongoing. There is a balance to be struck between the core skills and areas of practice of occupational therapy and the demands and duties of general team membership. In small teams, the occupational therapist is likely to be a core team member and will be expected to undertake thorough assessment of new referrals and to formulate and carry out a general treatment plan for the child, adolescent and their family, as well as be responsible for specific occupational therapy assessment and treatment. When working with adolescents, the focus is still on transitional roles, tasks and competencies, but it is less likely that the therapist will be able to work exclusively with this age group, and they will also need to develop the necessary skills to work with children and families. An example of how this works is shown in Figure 11.2.

The occupational therapist works mainly in the adolescent groups team. This team runs groups for adolescents aged 12–18 years, in vari[ous loca]tions including schools. The team also offers supervision and consultation for other workers running groups for young people both within the service and from other agencies.

Referrals are also made to the occupational therapist for specific individual work such as anxiety management. It is very common that young women who have been sexually abused will be referred for individual work. Gender considerations will apply because the young women usually ask for a female worker.

The occupational therapist is part of the family therapy team and offers assessment and treatment of families based on family therapy models. Specific further training is required for this.

WORKING CLOSELY WITH ADOLESCENTS

The demands on the therapist working with troubled adolescents are different from those of working with any other age group, not least because every therapist will have experienced an adolescence of their own. This brings a peculiar reality and resonance to the work, and can provoke surprising and powerful responses in the therapist. There is a variety and rapidity of reactions quintessential to adolescents that necessitate particular reciprocal behaviour. A therapist has to know how to work closely with adolescents in order to apply basic occupational therapy principles and skills to the work, something that Singh (1987) has called 'therapeutic bearing' – a way of being open and flexible yet boundaried and containing; curious and interested yet not intrusive; humorous and playful yet not mocking and dismissive; detached yet not indifferent; empathic yet not over-identified; enabling yet not overwhelming; separate and different yet not remote and clear and consistent yet not controlling.

It is not surprising that adolescents are naturally resistive to help and advice from adults, as one of their developmental tasks is to become emotionally independent from their parents. Some troubled adolescents actually live out the experience of that change by demanding closeness and intimacy and then fending off all offers of help. The change

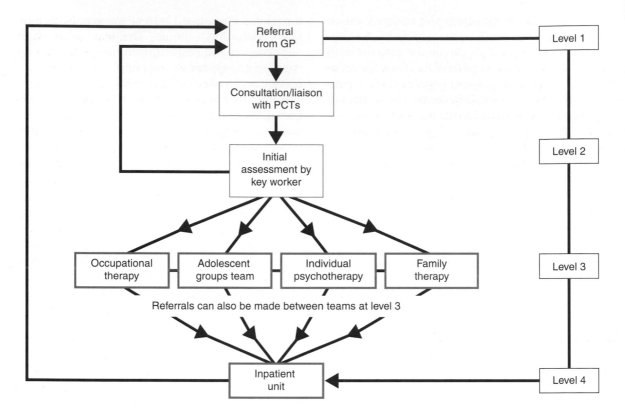

Occupational therapist could be:
- involved in consultation/liaison with PCTs
- key worker at Tier 2
- member of one or more teams at Tier 3
- member of inpatient team at Tier 4

Figure 11.2   Access routes from Tier 1 services provided by Exeter Child, Adolescent and Family Consultation Service.

between the two can be rapid and unpredictable. In order to remain responsive, the therapist will have to 'think on their feet' a lot of the time. This way they can be tolerant and flexible and not become equally resistive in return. A 'tit for tat' response to hostility is an unsafe way of working in adolescent therapy, as in the attitude: 'If you don't want my help, I can't be bothered either'. It is a common reaction of therapists who are rigid and unimaginative in their approach, and who are unaware that an indifferent response to their clients' distress can be interpreted as enmity.

Equally, troubled adolescents are often dismissive and verbally abusive to the therapist, for example 'You're crap, you're like my mother, you don't really care about me, you're only doing this because you get paid'. As a result, the therapist can feel useless, deskilled, and personally insulted and attacked. It is important to remember that the adolescent's behaviour is a reflection of their inner world and may be the only way they know of dealing with their internal distress, pain and confusion. Adolescents can display appalling behaviour without meaning to do so. The strong impact on the therapist is because the feelings are so real and intense. Managing this situation well requires a delicate balance between being relatively detached, so as not to take the behaviour personally, while remaining emotionally available and responsive. It is easy to become defensive and to be provoked into a parental response, and be either over-critical or over-caring.

For occupational therapists, who will be working to enhance self-esteem and efficacy, it is particularly relevant to acknowledge the adolescent's need for personal autonomy and recognition. However, when an adolescent is employing powerful rejecting manoeuvres it can be difficult to notice achievements, however small they may appear. The therapist can be trapped in a cycle of negative attention from which it is hard to break out. They can be seduced by rules and regulations and slip into thinking that is the only way of managing adolescent rebellion. It can be helpful to reframe superficially negative behaviour in a positive way (see Box 11.3).

It is generally agreed by most therapists in adolescent psychiatry that therapeutic interventions need to be of an active nature, rather than passive or interpretative. This is not an alien concept to occupational therapists. However, it can be difficult to engage an oppositional adolescent in any meaningful tasks or activities. Again, it is important to understand and acknowledge the underlying reasons for behaviour. Otherwise, the therapist can easily substitute insensitive mismanagement for empathy, which is not likely to foster engagement in any sort of activity, and the adolescent is likely to dismiss any task as trivial and worthless.

It is likely that many clients' difficulties are a result of adults misusing and abusing their position of power. Adults, particularly the significant ones such as parents and teachers, are potent role models in the lives of children and adolescents. They should be there to offer safe and containing boundaries yet increasing opportunities for the adolescent to experiment with ways of coping on their own. However, many adults have inappropriate boundaries, as in the case of sexual abuse.

Box 11.3 Case example: Jane

Jane, aged 15, left the unit without permission. Searches in the immediate vicinity failed to locate her. After 4 hours she returned, saying she had been to see her boyfriend. Staff praised her for getting herself back safely but clearly reiterated the rules regarding absences from the unit and explained the anxiety she had caused. Validation of her return rather than punishment of her absence was preferable in order to promote a sense of personal responsibility.

Therapists are significant adults within the context of their practice, and their behaviour and attitudes will be noticed and taken in by clients. Therapists are not only 'on trial' for their professional ability but for their ability to be an adult. Those new to working with adolescents can mistakenly believe that the best way of joining with clients is to identify with them by trying to be adolescent too. Clients rarely want therapists' reminiscences and re-enactments of their own adolescence. Nor do they want someone who demands respect and obedience simply for being older and more experienced. They want an adult who can face up to the challenge of confrontation in a containing, non-retaliatory way and who is secure in their personal identity and point of view. It is through that difference that adolescents can begin to explore and experiment with their own identity.

The job of the therapist is to work closely with and survive the specific challenges of the adolescent and not to be disappointed when they get no thanks or recognition for doing so. They need to remain flexible, tolerant and containing in their approach while thinking 'on their feet' in order to respond to unexpected behaviour, which could be positive or negative. They also need to remain aware of their own needs and feelings, and seek the appropriate ongoing support.

OCCUPATIONAL THERAPY ASSESSMENT

In adolescent psychiatry the occupational therapy assessment is usually a description of observed behaviours in order to ascertain the client's level of skills and competencies and to indicate the appropriate treatment. An adolescent does not function in isolation, so the assessment should also take account of important environmental factors such as family and school. Key adults in those settings may be able to provide information that the adolescent is unable or unwilling to supply. The family setting is particularly important because the expectations and pressures exerted in families can have both positive and negative effects. At best, they can provide encouragement and stimulation for achievement and a safe base from which to move on to adult roles and occupations. At worst, they can promote anxiety, anger, helplessness, apathy and withdrawal, all of which prevent adolescents from performing well and increase the likelihood of maintaining them in the sick role.

There are times when liaison with the family is contraindicated, for example when child protection issues are involved.

Before beginning the assessment it is also important to ascertain the following:

- any precautions that are necessary in approaching the client
- the client's developmental level
- any contract made on admission
- existing or previous involvement of other professionals
- any ongoing or previous child protection issues
- any legal issues (e.g. current court cases, divorce proceedings).

Methods of assessment

These are the main methods of assessment:

1. Specific observation
2. Personal interview
3. Standardised tests
4. Self-rating methods
5. Projective activities.

Each can be used in varying combinations depending on time available, the needs of the client, and the therapeutic orientation of the service.

Specific observation

Observation is a method of assessment that is continuous and often subconscious. It happens in both informal and formal ways. In the community, it is prohibitively time consuming and impractical to observe the adolescent in all their settings. Liaison with other professionals, such as teachers, and talking to the family are vital to obtain that information. On the inpatient unit there will be informal observations daily in the natural settings, such as milieu groups, leisure time with peers, meal times, in the school or educational environment. There are a myriad of behaviour patterns and emotions to observe. It is important to begin to recognise rele-

vant and important cues and develop the discipline and skills to record and report them accurately and specifically. This is not just for personal use but for that of colleagues. The accurate handover of information is vital for the safe and correct care of the clients, particularly in the inpatient setting, so it is important to develop good communication skills in handovers and case conferences.

For a more structured and specific observation it is useful to use a checklist. The benefits of a checklist are:

- It can be applied to many situations and tasks.
- It aids objectivity and reduces the effect of personal bias.
- Behaviour can be directly observed, not inferred.
- It can be graded and repeated, and so provides a record over time.
- It can be presented as an actual report to go into the case notes, which can easily be referred to by other professionals.

There are many checklist items to use, such as:

1. Personal presentation
2. Activity accomplishment
3. Group skills
4. Relationships with adults
5. Relationship with peers.

General items can be broken down into more specific definitions and each item or definition can be graded using a rating scale. For example, group skills could include:

- tolerance of others
- acceptance of rules
- level of participation.

The rating scale could be:

- A = no serious problems, likely to manage
- B = some problems, only moderate attainment
- C = considerable difficulty, needs further help.

An activity can be used as the focus for the observations. This helps to establish a therapeutic context and may be less threatening and more comfortable for the adolescent (Moll & Valiant Cook 1997). The type of activity should be recorded and dated so that it can be repeated at a later date and the results compared for evaluation.

Cooking is a particularly useful activity with adolescents because:

- there can be a quickly achieved end result, important for those whose concentration span is poor
- it is realistic and familiar so can be used with a variety of clients
- it is easy to grade (cooking a full meal is probably too elaborate for an assessment; simple cakes or biscuits are a better choice)
- seeing what happens to the end-result can be instructive. Does the adolescent
  - keep it to him or herself?
  - share it with the therapist or others?
  - take it home?
  - refuse to eat any of it? (not because it is inedible!)
  - destroy it?

Personal Interview

The aims are:

- to gain specific information about the client
- to initiate and/or develop the therapeutic relationship
- to explain the purpose and function of occupational therapy and how it will be part of an overall treatment plan
- to extend opportunities for observation and explore any observations previously made.

In the inpatient unit the adolescent will have many such interviews with a variety of staff, particularly on and near admission. It is very galling to be asked the same questions over and over again, and doing so guarantees non-response and hostility. Basic information can be collected from the medical notes. It is incumbent on the occupational therapist to make their interview relevant to their treatment aims, and of intrinsic interest to the adolescent. The Model of Human Occupation has much to offer here. The emphasis on roles and personal choice and meaning is particularly relevant to adolescents and the overall aims of occupational therapy treatment.

Skill and imagination are needed to make the questions suitable for each client. It may be

---

Box 11.4 Case example: Kate

Kate was 15 years old on admission. She had been anorectic for approximately 3 years and had been hospitalised on several occasions, both in paediatric wards and private clinics. She lived at home with her natural parents and two older brothers. Her father was a successful local businessperson and her mother was a housewife and partner in the business. Kate was described as an intelligent young woman who was expected to get A grades at GCSE. She was an accomplished artist and wanted to be a graphic designer.

When I met with Kate for assessment we used activity as a focus as she was nervous and hesitant, but also rather dismissive of the assessment procedure, owing to her previous admissions. I got the impression that she thought she could not be asked anything new, and she was practised at answering what she thought we all wanted to hear. She chose to make Fimo jewellery. The activity helped her to relax; she was familiar with the medium and she knew she could easily produce a good end-result.

In my questions I particularly put the emphasis on the meaning of activities to her. Did she do what she really enjoyed or did she only choose things she was good at in order to feel in control and efficacious? I asked her to identify the situations where she felt out of control and incompetent, and to describe how she coped. We talked about how her eating habits had interfered with her pursuit of activities and how her time had become governed by and structured around food and meal times. I asked her about friends and socialising, and whether she generally pursued activities alone or with others. We talked about her family and their expectations of her and how she felt this affected her illness. I asked her to identify her present and future roles.

---

appropriate to include questionnaires and checklists, or to focus on an activity (see Box 11.4).

Young people with anorexia nervosa are characterised as intelligent, high-achieving perfectionists who usually have a wide range of interests, particularly artistic and athletic. As their life becomes increasingly organised around food and the preoccupation with dieting and other methods of losing weight, the range and scope of their leisure activities gradually narrows and takes second place. They usually have a very low sense of self-esteem, which is reinforced by the unattainably high standards they set for themselves. They often come from middle class, controlling, high-achieving families, and there is now evidence to suggest that many mothers of anorectic daughters have had, or do have, an eating disorder themselves.

The assessment should reflect all the above issues. The clues to an appropriate treatment plan lie in the answers given.

Standardised tests

There are appropriate standardised tests available but most of them originate in the USA. Copies of tests can be difficult to obtain from publishers, but they do offer the best evaluative assessment because of the high degree of reliability and validity.

Self-rating methods

These assessments involve the completion of a questionnaire or rating scale. They are a beneficial tool with this age group because:

- the focus of attention is shifted away from the possible pressure of a one-to-one interview
- the adolescent is actively involved in the assessment
- the adolescent has the opportunity to give their own view of themselves
- they can facilitate communication. It may be easier to talk after, or while, writing.
- conversely, they can reduce the amount of talking needed and be suitable for clients who find verbal communication difficult.
- an enormous quantity of information can be gathered on one form. This may be preferable to asking a similar number of questions.

Questionnaries can seem dehumanising and make the adolescent feel they are worth no more than a few ticks (Finlay 1988). When compiling your own questionnaire, endeavour to design it, in both content and appearance, in a way that is appropriate and attractive to the target group. There could be different versions for different age groups, or one of the young people could contribute to the design.

Examples of relevant questionnaires are:

- anxiety rating scales
- roles questionnaire
- hobbies/interests questionnaire
- self-concept questionnaire.

Projective activities

Occupational therapists in the UK do not generally use formal projective tests (Finlay 1988). However, it is helpful to tap into unconscious material and so release emotions and reactions previously hidden. Projective activities are designed to explore these deeper feelings. Examples of the techniques used are:

- creative writing
- projective art
- drama therapy
- mime
- music therapy.

The techniques rely on the analysis and interpretation of the material presented. Sometimes this comes from the client and sometimes from the therapist. Interpretations made by the therapist should be posed to the client and not imposed on them. It is important to remember that all projective techniques should be used with discretion. The nature of unconscious material is a highly potent one and overinterpretation or misinterpretation can be misleading and damaging. Anyone using these techniques should have access to a supervisor who is properly qualified and experienced (Hagedorn 1997). Having said this, there are many exercises that access feelings in no better way. Examples are using clay, drawing, drama and creative writing.

Using clay.

- Make your family as people, objects, animals or symbols.
- Make your ideal family – how you would like them to be.
- Make a symbolic image of yourself.
- Make a clay island – give yourself a place to live; who else would be there with you? Would you try to escape?

Drawing.

- Where you wish you could be – an ideal place.
- Three wishes you would like to come true.
- A secret.
- How you see yourself/how others see you/how you would like to be seen.

Drama.

- Use objects in the room to sculpt your family and put yourself into the picture – you can use yourself or another object.
- Guided fantasy.

Creative writing.

- Write down a description of yourself as if it were being written by your best friend.

For many more useful exercises, see *Windows to Our Children* by Violet Oaklander (1978).

Assessment is not a procedure that is carried out in isolation from the rest of the therapeutic work. It marks the beginning of the therapeutic relationship. It is not possible to carry out an assessment without making therapeutic interventions. For example, it may be necessary to comment on or manage difficult behaviour, or to use a counselling technique to facilitate the assessment interview (see Box 11.5).

The fear of possible humiliation is very important to bear in mind when working with this age group. For an adolescent, the pain of losing face is an acute reality which can seem to an adult out of all proportion to the situation. To underestimate its potency could be detrimental to the therapeutic relationship.

During the assessment, the time spent with the adolescent and the accompanying attention paid to them may be the first time, for a long time, that their feelings and thoughts have been recognised. This process can create a fertile atmosphere in which they say more than they had intended or, equally, more than the therapist had been prepared to hear. This could mean a disclosure or part-disclosure of abuse. This is a disquieting prospect for many therapists. Should this happen, the important thing is not to panic and to listen calmly and attentively. Never promise confidentiality that cannot be kept and be open with the adolescent about what is going to happen to the disclosed information. Above all, consult with colleagues as to the best course of action and never try to manage such disclosures alone. At the same

---

Box 11.5 Case example: Nicola

Nicola was 13 years old when she was admitted. She was brought into the unit on a Section, which is relatively unusual for someone so young. For some months she had been withdrawing from her family and spending more and more time in her room. This was not worrying behaviour at first. However, Nicola stopped attending school and began refusing to eat until, finally, just before her admission, she had barricaded herself in her room and was refusing to come out. She was also cutting herself with razor blades.

When I first went to see her she was in the corner of her room with a blanket over herself, shouting obscenities, spitting at anyone who approached and refusing to talk. I had been qualified for about 2 months and Nicola was my first really uncooperative client. I decided to see her for a very brief time each day, just a few minutes, in order to reiterate who I was, to check how she was and to give her an opportunity to talk if she wanted to. I wanted to strike a balance between giving her some control and giving her clear and safe boundaries. After a few days she let me stay in the room without spitting or throwing things, but she still refused to talk. I remembered the counselling technique of mirroring the client's posture to try to ascertain their feelings. I discussed the idea with my colleagues and it was decided that I would try this with Nicola.

Next time I went to see her I sat quietly in the room and covered myself with a blanket. After a minute or so her curiosity overwhelmed her and she asked me what I was doing. I explained, and said it had given me some ideas as to why she may be behaving as she was. I described to her the feelings I was having sitting under the blanket. I was feeling in control and safe, yet scared and trapped into keeping the blanket over me for fear of losing face. I wondered if it was the same for her. Her reply is unrepeatable here but I knew some tension was broken and, in retrospect, this intervention did mark a turn in our relationship. When it was possible to begin a formal assessment I felt that some trust had already been established between us, and that Nicola was able to cooperate without feeling humiliated.

---

time, it is important to be aware of both local and service child protection procedures.

Once the assessment is complete and the information has been collated, organised in a coherent fashion and recorded, the next step is to decide who has access to the information. The issues of confidentiality and trust are paramount, particularly for adolescents.

Among colleagues, try to distinguish between those to whom the information is absolutely necessary, those to tell on a 'need to know' basis, and those who may be interested in the information but do not need to be informed. Then consider the needs of the adolescent and their family/carers.

Occupational therapy is based on the idea of purposeful activity and the client will be expected to be actively involved in the treatment process. A therapeutic relationship is founded on trust. In this client group many will already have had their trust abused by supposed caring and trusted adults. They will be especially alert and sensitive to possible deceptions. Being cagey and indirect about the conclusions of the assessment and the plans for future treatment is counterproductive. A degree of openness is a good foundation for therapeutic work and the client's cooperation and engagement.

A complicating factor is that the therapist is likely to be dealing with both the client and their family/carers. Ever present is the tension between adolescent autonomy and parental authority. The therapist has to take account of both. The involvement of parents/carers is not mandatory but advisable in most cases. With older adolescents, careful negotiation about the boundaries of confidentiality is particularly relevant because of different legal considerations. These issues are explored further in Chapter 15.

In some cases it may be helpful to make a therapeutic contract in a written form for the adolescent and their family or carers. It can be falsely assumed that an adolescent will appreciate what is required of them without explanation, and the contract is a reminder and a boundary for all concerned. It is useful to refer back to the contract in periods of tension or confusion in the ongoing therapy.

OCCUPATIONAL THERAPY TREATMENT

The main focus of occupational therapy interventions is to help the adolescent acquire the skills and competencies that will enhance their ability to cope with the maturational tasks of adolescence and so progress to adulthood. For troubled adolescents it is these tasks that are being experienced as disturbing and disabling (Singh 1987).

There is an abundance of written material elsewhere on treatment planning, setting aims and objectives, and activity analysis which can be universally applied to this client group, so the emphasis will be on specific interventions.

Therapeutic interventions

Occupational therapists have a wide range of interventions for adolescents and their families/carers. These are shown in Box 11.6.

This chapter does not allow for a detailed description of everything listed. However, in both inpatient and community settings the predominant intervention for occupational therapist is group work, so this is the focus here.

Group work

Adolescents grow up in naturally occurring groups such as family, school and friends. In these groups a sense of trust in the world develops, a personal and social identity is formed, and mutual support is offered. The nature and quality of these interpersonal relationships is an important factor in the psychological health of the child, adolescent and, eventually, the adult. It is known that if chil-

---

Box 11.6 The range of interventions used by an occupational therapist working with adolescents

Individual	Group	Family
Self-care skills	Social/interpersonal and life skills	Individual consultation with parent
Social/interpersonal and life skills	Problem-solving skills	Joint sessions with parent(s) and adolescent
Problem-solving skills	Leisure/work skills	
Leisure/work skills	Anxiety management	
Anxiety management	Creative/self expression	
Creative/self expression	Projective techniques	
Projective techniques	Milieu groups (inpatient)	
Counselling	Problem-oriented (e.g. bereavement, eating disorders, sexual abuse)	
	Psychotherapy (talking only)	
	Parent support	

dren do not acquire the skills to relate well to their peers the likelihood of psychological disorder in adolescence and adulthood is greatly increased.

Group work is an attractive form of therapy for adolescents because it provides an opportunity for them to be actively involved and give and share their opinions and feelings with others. This resembles behaviour in their own naturally occurring peer groups. Other interventions, such as family therapy, can feel more adult oriented and dominated.

All groups with adolescents will have an educational component as they learn more about themselves in relation to others as well as specific coping skills. Box 11.7 summarises the benefits of using group work.

In order to run any group, the therapist requires a knowledge of group dynamics. This is concerned with how groups function and includes the factors that influence the interaction of group members, and the developmental stages of the group. Figure 11.3 shows the structural properties of a group that aid its functioning.

This chapter does not allow for more than a simple explanation of group dynamics. For more information, see Further reading.

The group leader

Adolescent groups need a structured setting with an emphasis on containment, support and positive regard rather than the interpretation of feelings and actions. The leader's task is to keep a balance between the three elements shown in Figure 11.3. The therapist in an adolescent group is much more likely to be challenged about their leadership role than in an adult group. There are also likely to be more challenges about the setting of boundaries and limits. These challenges can come, for example, in the form of personal attacks on the leader or by actions such as persistently arriving late to the group. The motive behind the challenges is often to provoke the leader into hostile behaviour that reinforces the adolescent's negative view of adults (see Box 11.8). A wise leader stays calm, avoids being seduced into retaliatory behaviour, is directive and active, and gives feedback that is reality

---

Box 11.7 The benefits of groupwork

Why group work?

1. It allows the individual to make maximum use of peer learning.
2. It can increase a person's knowledge of social behaviour and social skills.
3. Positive contributions will receive recognition. Recognition can help a person achieve self-confidence and self-actualisation.
4. Receiving feedback may also accelerate a person's learning and results.
5. It makes a sense of belonging and mutual support through shared experience.
6. It makes beneficial use of group pressure (e.g. for attitude change).
7. Research shows that group work can offer faster and more permanent change, especially social change, than individual interventions.
8. It offers an opportunity to use initiative and planning skills, and individuals are thus able to practise self-control.

Why groups for adolescents?

1. Acceptance by virtue of similar experience
2. Reduced feelings of isolation
3. Support from others who have had similar experience
4. Provision of a predictable, regular and safe environment away from home
5. A supportive place to explore feelings and thoughts
6. A chance to invest in new relationships
7. A chance to explore new ways of coping, develop new skills and attain a sense of mastery over situations

Yalom's curative factors in group psychotherapy (Yalom 1975)

1. Imparting information
2. Instillation of hope
3. Universality
4. Altruism
5. The corrective recapitulation of the family group
6. Developing of socialising techniques
7. Imitative behaviour
8. Interpersonal learning
9. Group cohesiveness
10. Catharsis
11. Existential factors

---

based and relatively concrete and in a form that the adolescent can use and understand.

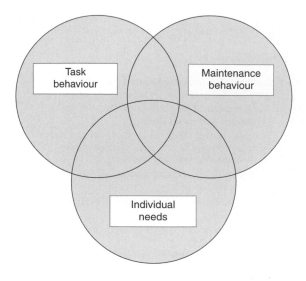

1. Task behaviour helps the team define and carry out the task.
2. Maintenance behaviour helps the group maintain work as a team and is concerned with group needs.
3. Individual needs is concerned with individual members of the group. If one person's needs become too prominent they may interfere with the work of the group.

These elements are interdependent and should be kept in balance.

Figure 11.3 Structural properties of a group.

Setting up the group

Box 11.9 shows the necessary considerations when setting up a group. While these considerations can be applied universally to all group situations, there are some that prevail when working with adolescents.

Type of group. For adolescents there are benefits to an open group. Members can join and leave at various points depending on assessment and evaluation. Throughout the life of the group, regular reviews can be held for each member with their family/carers when an end date can be set or more sessions offered. The advantage is that the leaders can respond quickly to referrals and offer further work when it is needed. However, an open group is a big commitment for the leaders, who have to 'diary space' well into the future.

Choosing a co-therapist. It is preferable to run a group with someone else. It is unlikely that that person will be another occupational therapist in

Box 11.8 Case example: interpersonal skills group

In an interpersonal skills group for year 10 pupils in a secondary school, the challenge was about whether or not participants should be allowed to smoke during the break. The group was run off-site by a male teacher from the school and myself. In the shared task of establishing the group rules, the leaders made the mistake of not making the no-smoking rule non-negotiable. This was done in a naive belief that this would be an imposition and not negotiation, and therefore contrary to the therapeutic notion of empowerment. What ensued was a battle for control of the group, especially aimed at the teacher.

For two of the group members it was important to 'rubbish' the group by making it seem no different from the classroom environment and so to provoke the teacher into replicating the hostile behaviour they had previously encountered from other teachers. He was temporarily drawn into retaliatory behaviour by being similarly aggressive.

As a non-teacher I was temporarily immune from the challenge and so could observe yet remain detached from the situation. This enabled me to recognise and label the fears behind the challenge for the group, whilst owning that a mistake had been made by the therapists. In future groups the no-smoking rule was made clear and mandatory at the beginning. We were seduced into acting as though running the group off-site meant that none of the usual school rules applied. This compromised the position of the teacher and consequently both of us as group leaders – a fact instinctively exploited by the group members.

this area of work. It is important to choose a fellow therapist carefully. Co-therapy has often been compared to a marriage. Leaders should enjoy working together and be able to work out differences between them in the group in a way that offers a good model of conflict resolution. They need to take time to get to know each other and to learn about and accept differences in personal style and professional bias. In mixed groups for adolescents it is usually advisable to have a male and female co-therapist. This provides role models for both genders and a replication of parental figures.

In Yalom's curative factors in group psychotherapy (see Box 11.7), one of the factors cited is the corrective recapitulation of the family group. For many troubled adolescents their experience of family life is abusive and distressing. They have poor real or internalised models of family relationships. To witness adults behaving in a safe way and by joining in with the group's thera-

Box 11.9 Factors to consider when planning a group

Type of group	Open or closed
Theoretical base	Does the group fit in with service philosophy?
Method	Drama
	Projective techniques
	Role play
Group leaders	How many?
	Who?
	Gender mix?
	What roles will they have?
	Style of leadership
Supervision	Who will do it?
	How often?
	When?
Where will group take place?	What rooms are necessary?
How long will it last?	Length of whole group
	Length of each session
	How frequently will group meet?
	At what time of day?
Method of referral	Advertising the group beforehand
	Is referral form needed?
	What feedback will referrers get?
How will group members be selected?	Age
	Gender
	By identified problem (e.g. eating disorder)
	What assessment is necessary?
Parents/carers	Are they involved?
	How are they informed about the group?
How many will be in the group?	
What resources are needed?	Transport
	Materials
Recording	How and where will sessions be recorded?
Evaluation	Is it possible?
	Will other professionals be needed?

peutic culture they are able to begin to build a new symbolic 'family', one where needs and wishes are taken care of and fears and worries can be worked through and resolved.

Transport arrangements. In groups for adolescents the issue of transport is an important one. It may be necessary to liaise with hospital transport or taxi firms, or to make arrangements with parents or carers. For adolescents below a certain age, drivers may not agree to provide transport without an escort, or may refuse to accept previously disruptive or aggressive passengers. As community groups often include members from a wide geographical area, it may be practical and convenient to transport two or more group members together. However, this may set up an unhelpful and destructive subgroup within the

group, and make it necessary to choose between pragmatic and process considerations.

Giving the group a title. The way in which a group is advertised, titled and presented to an adolescent is significant. Because of the core aims of treatment, occupational therapists will be expected to run social skills groups. But adolescents may be put off by a group with this title. In the outpatient groups team to which the writer belongs, the team has abandoned titles and has groups for younger and older adolescents only. These are activity-based groups open to adolescents of similar age with varying problems, including poor interpersonal skills. The activities are an eclectic mix of drama games, discussion and creative techniques. These activities are adapted and applied to the varying needs of the group members, because in

Box 11.10 Case example: age range in the group

In a group for young women aged 14–16 years who had been sexually abused, the leaders were referred someone aged 13 who had been sexually abused by her father, who was at present serving a prison sentence for the offence. She had said to her social worker that she wanted to meet other girls who had had similar experiences. She had not had any previous individual therapy. Her mother was very keen for her to attend and put a lot of pressure on her daughter to agree to go to the group.

The group needed one or two more members to be able to run. The leaders were reluctant to take her because of her age: the other group members were all 16 or nearly 16. But the leaders were seduced by the girl's apparent enthusiasm to join and their need for another member. It was difficult to convene such groups more than once a year and they did not want to disappoint the existing members. So she joined. It was a mistake. That 3-year age gap was apparent from the first session, and the girl immediately became the youngest sister. The other young women were coping with boyfriends and exams, and she was still playing with dolls.

Despite the best efforts of the therapists the girl chose to leave the group. This left the other young women with unnecessary feelings of guilt and responsibility, and left her unable to access any other form of therapy. The therapists learnt a painful but important lesson about sticking to good group-work practice.

groups where activity is the focus the end-result may be less important than the process of the group and what individuals learn about themselves and their relationships with others.

Parents/carers.   Parents or carers can feel isolated when their child is receiving therapeutic help. This may lead to rivalrous behaviour towards the therapist and possible sabotage of the therapy by not cooperating with transport arrangements or continually making alternative appointments for their child to coincide with the group. To minimise this, it is vital to liaise with parents or carers and give them some information in general terms while respecting the confidentiality of the group. It may be necessary to set up a simultaneous support group for parents or to have regular reviews throughout the life of the group. This will have implications for the number of professionals needed to run and support the group endeavour.

Timing.   The timing of the group is significant. Parents usually request an after-school time, while adolescents are often only too happy to miss lessons. If there are to be breaks in the group, try to make them coincide with school holidays. Many families go away then and adolescents tend to correlate holiday time with time off, so there are likely to be many group absences. It is also best to avoid exam time such as GCSEs and A levels.

Group membership.   The membership of a group has a powerful effect on the interactions that occur (see Box 11.10) and can enhance or impede its progress. It is important to choose members with group effectiveness in mind. Box 11.11 shows the factors that need to be considered.

Box 11.11 Factors to be considered when selecting members for a group

Motivation to attend	Adolescents may attend to please adults (e.g. parents). The last say should be with the adolescent as to whether they want to join or not
Age and developmental level	Keep the age band narrow: 2 years between oldest and youngest. An older but emotionally undeveloped adolescent may feel more comfortable with a younger age group
Sex	Mixed or single sex groups
Ability to communicate	Participants need to be able to verbalise feelings and thoughts adequately
Degree of disturbance	An adolescent experiencing psychotic thought is not likely to function well in a group
Behavioural difference	It is useful to include adolescents with a variety of difficulties as this increases the repertory of skills and interests available to the group and encourages sharing and modelling. It is not a good idea to have a preponderance of members with uncontrolled aggression
Ability to relate to others	Consider levels of dependency, empathy and how an individual manages challenge and distress

From Benson 1997.

Managing the group

There is more to running a group than preparation, setting aims and objectives, and having detailed, well thought out session plans with developmentally appropriate activities. Inevitably, events will not happen according to plan and the therapist will need to be prepared to adapt to the actual behaviour in the group and to deviate from the prescribed programme. An understanding of group dynamics is crucial in order to explain what is happening and to inform the right intervention. Supervision is mandatory, even for experienced group therapists. The insight that can be provided by an impartial third person is invaluable (see Box 11.12).

Group endings

The endings of groups are often not as carefully thought out and planned for as the beginnings. The adolescents involved have often already experienced rejection, abuse, failure and abandonment by parents, peers and teachers.

Box 11.12 Case example: Darren

The members of an inpatient group all had poor social and interpersonal skills. The aim was to develop enough appropriate skills to enable the group to go together for a coffee in town. Behavioural principles were used with rehearsal, video feedback and role play. Darren was a 16-year-old with a history of psychotic illness, now well controlled by medication but with residual poor interpersonal skills and low tolerance of stress. The first time the video was used, he became very excited and high, and proceeded to take out his penis and wave it in front of the camera, much to the horror and consternation of myself and the rest of the group. I got embarrassed, panicked and asked him to leave the group, knowing that was punitive of Darren but not being able to think of anything else.

In my next supervision session my supervisor suggested I should have remembered the purpose of the group and used that as a basis to get the rest of the group to help me by saying: 'Is this what we want Darren to do when we go for a coffee?'. Afterwards I should have worked with the group to help Darren gain insight into the inappropriateness of his behaviour and help him to develop alternative ways of managing.

Therefore, endings will be especially significant for them. Near the end of groups, the hostility and challenge of the earlier stages may re-emerge. The therapist needs to be prepared. Groups do not heal all ills and even the best prepared for and executed endings leave members feeling abandoned and wanting more. The therapist will also have to leave knowing and acknowledging this sense of non-completion.

CONCLUSION

The likelihood is that most troubled adolescents go on to lead productive and fulfilling adult lives, but it is doubtful that therapists will ever see their clients as adults. They can be left wondering if their interventions had any long-lasting effects and how the mixture of therapeutic input and maturational forces has influenced the adolescent and their future. Occasionally, the therapist is lucky enough to get some feedback.

In the process of writing this chapter I was unexpectedly contacted by Elizabeth and Caroline, now aged 23 and 25 years respectively. I had worked with them for a period of 3–4 years as both inpatients and outpatients, when they were very difficult and disturbed young women, and the prognosis was poor for their managing adult life successfully. Now they had just returned from 18 months travelling round the world. Elizabeth was in her first term of a law degree and Caroline was training to be a counsellor.

Therapy is a complex yet subtle skill, perhaps never more so than in working with adolescents. Many of the values, beliefs and skills of occupational therapists are not obvious to the uninformed observer. The music hall image of 'baskets and bunnies' does much to undermine and devalue the profession. The following case material (see Box 11.13) demonstrates how occupational therapists, working with adolescents, have to consider many things concurrently on different levels, and illustrates the truth of Fleming's comment: 'Although what they do looks simple, what they know is often quite complex' (Fleming 1994, p. 24).

Box 11.13 Case example: Karen and Andrew

Karen and Andrew were involved in a cooking group. Karen was a young woman aged 15, with a history of intrafamilial sexual and physical abuse, chronic solvent abuse, cutting and overdosing. Andrew, a young man also aged 15, had a history of depression and antisocial behaviour following the acrimonious divorce of his parents. The aim of the group was to plan and cook a meal to which each member could invite one other person, staff or client.

During the preparation, Andrew enquired whether he could ask me a personal question, which was how he frequently started awkward conversations. My usual reply was that he could, but I may not agree to answer. He looked apprehensive and said: 'You're very flat-chested, aren't you?' Karen giggled nervously in the anticipation of my reply. I resisted an angry response due to personal embarrassment and asked A. why he was so concerned about my physical appearance. The ensuing conversation incorporated worries they both had about physical, personal and sexual identity, being attractive to the opposite sex, making friends, anger with their parents and fears for the future. We discussed how Andrew had started this conversation and how this may contravene my professional and personal boundaries and what less desirable outcomes may occur if he said similar things to other adults. We talked while continuing with the preparation of the meal and sat down at the end of 2 hours to lasagne and chocolate mousse, if I remember correctly.

REFERENCES

Anderson R, Dartington A (eds) 1998 Facing it out: clinical perspectives on adolescent disturbance. Duckworth, London
Benson J F 1997 Working more creatively with groups. Routledge, London
Conger J J, Petersen A C 1984 Adolescence and youth psychological development in a changing world, 3rd edn. Harper & Row, New York
Davis J 1990 Youth and the condition of Britain: images of adolescent conflict. Athlone Press, London
Davis M, Wallbridge D 1981 Boundary and space: an introduction to the work of D W Winnicott. H Karnac, London
Finlay L 1988 Occupational therapy practice in psychiatry. Croom Helm, London
Fleming M H 1994 The search for tacit knowledge. In: Mattingly C, Fleming M H (eds) Clinical reasoning: forms of inquiry in a therapeutic practice. F A Davis, Philadelphia, p 22
Franckel R 1998 The adolescent psyche: Jungian and Winnicottian perspectives. Routledge, London
Hagedorn R 1997 Foundations for practice in occupational therapy, 2nd edn. Churchill Livingstone, New York
Havighurst R J 1972 Development tasks and education, 3rd edn. McKay, New York
Jezzard R 1994 Adolescent psychotherapy. In: Clarkson P, Pokorny M (eds) A handbook of psychotherapy. Routledge, London, Part III, ch 10, p 195
Marchant M 1987 An introduction to adolescence. National Council of Voluntary Child Care, London
Moll S, Valiant Cook J 1997 'Doing' in mental health practice: therapists' beliefs about why it works. American Journal of Occupational Therapy 51(8): 662–670
NHS Health Advisory Service 1986 Bridges over troubled waters – a report on services for disturbed adolescents. NHS HAS, London
Oaklander V 1978 Windows to our children. Real People Press, Moab, Utah
Singh N 1987 Therapeutic work with in patient adolescents. Journal of Adolescence 10(2):119–131
Yalom I D 1975 The theory and practice of group psychotherapy. Basic Books, New York

FURTHER READING

Bain O, Sanders M 1990 Out in the open. A guide for young people who have been sexually abused. Virago Press, London

Bayard R T, Bayard J 1984 Help I've got a teenager! A survival guide for desperate parents. Exley Publications, Watford, UK

Dwivedi K N (ed) 1993 Group work with children and adolescents a handbook. Jessica Kingsley, London

Fisher N 1994 Your pocket guide to sex. Penguin, London

Gordon J, Grant G (eds) 1997 How we feel. An insight into the emotional world of teenagers. Jessica Kingsley, London

Lane D A, Miller A 1992 Child and adolescent therapy – a handbook. Open University Press, Buckingham

Preston-Shoot M 1987 Effective groupwork. Macmillan Education, Basingstoke

Stock Whitacker D 1985 Using groups to help people. Routledge, London

Varma V P (ed) 1992 The secret life of vulnerable children. Routledge, London

Occupational therapy in CAMHS internationally

SECTION CONTENTS

The context of CAMHS and the influences on therapeutic practice reflect the national health policies and the dominant frames of reference used by the profession. It is interesting to compare the development of occupational therapy in the USA, described by Laurette Olson in Chapter 12, with that in New Zealand as developed by Ann Christie and Rowena Scaletti in Chapter 13. Both these chapters demonstrate an awareness of the effects of ethnicity on the delivery of treatment programmes.

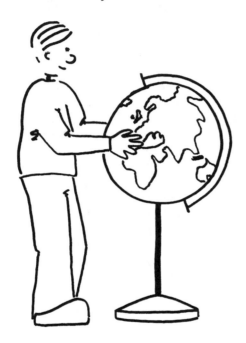

12

Child psychiatry in the USA

Laurette J. Olson

INTRODUCTION

Presently, only a small group of occupational therapists in the United States work with children with emotional disorders. In a survey done by the American Occupational Therapy Association (AOTA) in 1990, 9.2% of all occupational therapists reported working in mental health settings. Only 14.8% of that small group of therapists stated that they worked with clients under the age of 19 years. Some 20% of all occupational therapists in the United States surveyed in 1995 stated that they worked in school-based settings. Only 1.2% of these therapists reported working with children who exhibit serious emotional disorders. The reasons why so few therapists work with this population of children is not because children in the United States rarely experience psychiatric disorders. Funding for services such as occupational therapy for these children has been limited in comparison to the funding and job opportunities for occupational therapists to work with children with learning disabilities or physical dysfunction. In spite of this, occupational therapists have described dynamic practice working with children with mental illness and their families in a variety of settings (Florey & Greene 1997, Olson, 1999, Olson, Heaney & Soppas-Hoffman 1989, Schultz 1992). A growing number of therapists in the United States work with young children who exhibit symptoms of sensory integration disorders along with a vulnerability to developing emotional and behaviour disorders.

To describe the state and direction of occupational therapy in child and adolescent psychiatry in the United States, one must first examine its context. Occupational therapy is currently in a state of self-reflection owing to the changing landscape of health care in the United States. For-profit and not-for-profit health management companies now play a very active role in health-care provision, and health providers must provide daily data to company representatives in order for health coverage to commence or continue. Shortened lengths of hospital stays and brief outpatient treatments have occurred as health insurance companies focus on efficiency of service and profits. This has led health professionals to use assessments and treatments that are rapid and address acute, immediate needs for which managed-care companies are most likely to pay. Looking more carefully at the full range of needs that clients may have is not encouraged since this might require longer and more intensive intervention. Within this healthcare atmosphere, there has been a greater call within the profession for occupational therapists to seek employment in community-based practice settings where longer-term intervention that can potentially focus on improving the quality of everyday life of clients can occur. This is a practice setting in which occupational therapy will probably flourish in the 21st century.

Within this context, the profession of occupational therapy is renewing its allegiance to its core values and roots in the interest of occupational therapy's survival and continued growth in the twenty-first century. There has been a call for occupational therapists to address again the psychosocial needs of their clients as occupational therapists did earlier in the twentieth century. The leaders in occupational therapy education and practice are strongly advocating that occupational therapists focus on occupation as opposed to focusing primarily on underlying performance components (Fisher 1998, Trombly 1995, Wood 1995). Educational programmes are redesigning their curricula to reflect this shift in thinking. In the past, it was common practice for many occupational therapists primarily to assess and treat performance components. It was expected that, if clients had the underlying skills to perform activities, they could be successful in their daily occupations. This bottom-up approach led to more technical treatment that failed to distinguish occupational therapists from other professionals, as well as lessening occupational therapists' emphasis on helping persons develop and participate in occupations that were meaningful to them. At the same time, other professions have been struggling to incorporate daily function into their professional entities since managed-care companies have tied reimbursement to some functional measures. The leaders of the field of occupational therapy in the United States see the survival of the profession as tied to the profession's ability to renew its own belief in the power of occupation and then to articulate this to clients and those who fund services.

In AOTA's position paper on occupation (AOTA 1995), occupations were defined as: 'goal-directed pursuits which typically extend over time, have meaning to the performer and involve multiple tasks . . . occupations are the ordinary and familiar things that people do every day'. Fisher (1998, p. 511) has articulated an action-oriented definition of occupational therapy: 'enabling clients to seize, take possession of or occupy the spaces, time and roles of their lives'. The goal of an occupational therapist is to help clients use time and their environments to use or create opportunities for activity in a personally meaningful way that leads to their successful participation in their occupational roles. For children, occupations include participating in school work, structured and unstructured peer group activities, and family maintenance (i.e. eating with family members, completing household and self-care activities under their parents' supervision) and leisure activities. Their roles include being a student, a friend, a player, a son or daughter, a worker.

A client-centred top-down approach to occupational assessment and intervention is presently considered best practice by occupational therapy leaders in the United States. Understanding clients' occupational history, who they are in the context of their family, community and culture, and what their goals are for the future is the first step in the evaluation process. In working with children, this may include completing a play history with children's care-givers (Takata 1974) or discussing with children or their care-givers what the children's current interests and activities are and what goals each holds for the future. After gathering these data, therapists examine how clients participate in their daily occupations. Children might be observed playing soccer with peers or participating in classroom activities. Informal observations or tools such as the School Function Assessment (Coster 1997) may be used at this level of assessment. After analysing clients' strengths and difficulties in performing occupations, therapists may decide that, in order to assist that client to participate more successfully in occupational roles, they need to examine underlying performance components. After observing a child playing with peers or participating in educational tasks, a therapist may note signs that the child's ability to cope with challenges inherent in tasks or in interaction with others may be interfering with occupational performance. The therapist may use the Coping Skill Inventory (Zeitlin 1985) as a method specifically to analyse the child's coping skills.

Within the context of what has been described as best practice in the United States, I will describe what I understand to be optimal occupational therapy practice in child and adolescent psychiatry. I have come to my professional opinion through my own clinical work, research, and supervision of other occupational therapists and students. To make this chapter most understandable, the information about occupational therapy practice is divided according to critical performance component deficits that are typically noted as a therapist observes children with mental illness go about their daily occupations. Although these deficits must be understood within the context of children's occupations and should first be identified within the context of occupations, it is less repetitive and clearer to present the information under the headings of performance components.

COPING SKILLS

In observing children with emotional disorders, a striking barrier that these children typically exhibit is poor coping skills when confronted with challenges in activity and in interactions with others. Their coping strategies tend to be rigid instead of flexible, sometimes passive as opposed to active, and frequently unproductive. Although destroying a project, yelling at a teacher, or withdrawing from an assigned task without asking for help leads to reprimand and school failure, some children continually use these methods to cope with their frustration. Analysing children's or adolescents' strengths and deficits relative to coping is central to understanding how to help them manage the stresses inherent in participating in the everyday occupations of their developmental age. Working without a guide for such an analysis can make this a very overwhelming and frustrating task for the evaluating therapist. Children with mental illness typically exhibit significant, and at times pervasive, coping deficits which seem to blot out any awareness of their coping strengths.

A useful tool which may strengthen a therapist's ability to analyse coping behaviour, and may also serve as a guide for intervention, is the Coping Skill Inventory (Zeitlin 1985). To complete the Observation Form of the Coping Skills Inventory, a therapist observes identified children participating their everyday occupations over a period of time. The therapist then rates behaviours related to coping with oneself and with the environment on a five-point scale from not effective to consistently effective across situations. After completing the inventory, scores are derived for coping productivity, passive to active approaches, and rigid to flexible approaches relative to coping with the environment as well as with the self. The therapist graphs the scores so that one can visually see the areas of coping strength versus coping deficit. In addition, the guidelines for the inventory structure therapists to list children's most adaptive coping behaviours and the least adaptive behaviours. Therapists can then begin prioritising what would be most beneficial to address for individual children, consciously to foster children's use of their most adaptive coping behaviours in activity while developing areas of weakness. What therapists learn about children's coping styles and abilities can then be applied to all occupationally based interventions. To learn more about applying a coping frame of reference, it is recommended that readers peruse the work of Williamson & Szczepanski (1999).

The example given in Box 12.1 will hopefully make the use of the Coping Skills Inventory clear.

PARENT–CHILD INTERACTION

Of all of the occupational roles of childhood, being a child within a family is the most important role for most children. Strong parent–child relationships are important for healthy psychosocial development. The research based upon Mary Ainsworth's seminal work (1967) emphasises the relationship between a secure parent–child relationship and competence in childhood. Studies have correlated security in a parent–child relationship with peer competence, resilience, curiosity and prosocial behaviours (Arend, Gore & Sroufe 1979, Greenberg, Speltz & DeKlyen 1993, Waters, Wittman & Sroufe 1979). In a longitudinal study of a group of children from birth through adolescence, Murphy (1962) found that the most important factors in children's development of good coping skills was the quality of parents' enjoyment of their children

Box 12.1 Case example: Tommy

Tommy, a 9-year-old boy who was hospitalized for depression and a conduct disorder, demonstrated relatively active and slightly more productive coping behaviour when dealing with others in occupations such as group games with peers and cooking with his mother than when he participated in singular occupations. He exhibited more passive, less productive and rigid behaviour in individual occupations such as constructional play activities or doing his schoolwork. He exhibited good gross motor and fine motor skills and had a high energy level and enthusiasm for group activities. Some of the coping behaviours related to self that he specifically exhibited were rarely asking for help, using a very limited range of strategies to achieve goals, being closed to new ideas, not accepting of substitutes when his strategy did not work, and not bouncing back from disappointment in an activity.

After completing the Coping Skills Inventory, the therapist first reflected on the differences in Tommy's behaviour in peer and family activities versus his behaviour in parallel task activities. In group activities, Tommy was more of a follower and imitated the behaviour of others. He did not need to ask for help because he easily copied good models that were available within a group activity or allowed another to complete challenging parts of an activity. He was not often challenged by another person in any activity.

To develop Tommy's coping skills in deficit areas, his relative strength as a group participant was used. Since he exhibited the necessary underlying motor skills, motivation for activity and physical energy for activity, he could be challenged in an activity as long as others could take the lead in confronting challenges and problem-solving. When Tommy was not singled out, he maintained his composure, in spite of group challenges, to create new games and to build model planes in teams. All group members were encouraged to offer help to others and to ask for help as needed. The leader modelled and supported playful experimentation with activity ideas and approaches to tasks, as well as problem-solving out loud when confronted with a challenge. Over the course of a few groups, Tommy began to offer his ideas and tentatively participated in working out those ideas.

In a parent–child activity group, Tommy was offered open-ended projects; he and his mother were supported and guided by a therapist as they created sculptures and toys from scrap materials. They built a boat and a robot from boxes and styrofoam; created puppets from papier mâché, tin foil and tape. As she saw her son succeed and exhibit pleasure in activity with her, Tommy's mother began to cue him in a manner similar to the therapist.

and parents' active support and encouragement of them (Fig. 12.1).

Through the parent–child relationship, children first experience play and learn to interact socially to gain attention, approval and help. If parent–child relationships are strong and interactions regular, consistent and typically positive, children expect positive attention and approval when they seek it in an appropriate way. Children feel confident that, if they need help or support, their parents will be available. This provides a sense of calmness and security as children face the challenges of everyday life. If children are not confident or do not expect support and assistance as they need it, they will more likely feel overwhelmed by challenges and be less willing to confront those challenges.

When children have mental illness, it is not uncommon to have parents report primarily negative interactions with their children and few, if any, pleasurable activity interactions. Attentional difficulties, inability to contain impulses, obsessions, compulsions, delusions or withdrawal from reality will challenge even the most positive and supportive care-givers. Parents may spend their time with their mentally ill children trying to contain problem behaviour; they may be very overwhelmed and feel unsuccessful in managing and helping their child to function in everyday activities. It may be difficult to experience enjoyment in interacting with these children and negative cycles of interaction may develop which limit parents' ability to offer these children support and encouragement. Some parents may actively avoid interacting with their children once their children are calm. Others may feel negative or angry toward their children and have difficulty recognizing positive behaviours that their children exhibit.

Adult behaviour plays a significant role in some children's development of mental illness; some parents may be physically or sexually abusive to their children or neglect their offspring. Parents may also have their own psychiatric disorders which may limit their capacity to parent. They may also be struggling with multiple life stressors including poverty, homelessness, divorce or spousal abuse. Their children may be left angry or withdrawn, or they may imitate the maladaptive behaviours that they observe in their parents. This may limit children's ability to engage and interact successfully with other care-givers in their lives. If children cannot attract care-givers positively they are not likely to receive the emotional nurturance or the opportunities they need to learn occupational behaviour from care-givers.

While there are ample professionals to focus on the problems that bring a family to a treatment centre and to educate family members on managing the mental illness, there are fewer professionals who focus on facilitating positive activity interaction between parents and children. Positive activity interaction with significant others in one's life provides a person with the energy to deal with conflicts and problems when they arise with these significant others. It is as important to deal with the lack of positive activity involvement in families that include a member who is mentally ill as it is to decrease the negative interaction. Occupational therapists are well qualified professionals to deal with this issue. Families can be helped to use activities as a means to promote positive feelings and pleasurable interactions among themselves. Learning to figure out how to build a kite, playing a cooperative game, preparing a meal together can build family camaraderie and a sense of connectedness, as well as promote problem-solving skills.

Parent–child activity groups

One way that occupational therapists have applied these ideas in psychiatric settings is

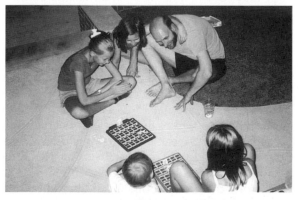

Figure 12.1   A father enjoying a board game.

through the development of parent–child activity groups. Such groups have been used in both inpatient and community settings, and with parents and their children of varied ages (Olson 1999, Olson et al 1989). Concepts of group theory (Yalom 1975), occupational therapy theory (Fidler & Fidler 1978, Reilly 1974) and parent–child interaction research and theory (Heard 1981, Murphy 1962, Murphy & Moriarty 1976) have been used as a theoretical base for these groups. A parent–child activity group is a multifamily group in which everyday constructional activities, tabletop or gross motor games, or play are used as a concrete means to engage individual family members with one another in a manner that they would likely perceive as pleasurable and positive. As other families are also present and participating in activities with their own members, there is an opportunity to learn from them via observation, as well as through interaction.

A parent–child activity group typically consists of four to seven families and two group leaders who facilitate and support individual parent–child activity and overall group interaction. The leaders introduce activities, assist families in adapting activities, and monitor group and individual family dynamics. In addition to fostering more frequent, positive and developmentally supportive interaction between parents and their children, these groups are also useful in assessing the quality of parent–child interaction in everyday leisure occupations.

Use of activity

Constructional play is frequently used to engage parents with their children. It is play activity in which children build from their own imagination for no other purpose other than the pleasure derived from the activity. It is one of the most effective types of play to develop concentration, problem-solving and imagination in children (Sylva 1984). By the nature of the challenges presented by construction for children, parents have frequent opportunities to help, guide, make suggestions and praise their children. The leaders help parents through offering suggestions or concretely showing a parent how to manipulate

materials in a way that might help a child to enact a plan. A leader might help a family problem-solve by talking through a problem and a potential plan with them. Other families that are present serve as role models, sources of ideas for projects, and often offer concrete help. It is important that the leaders support each family sufficiently to ensure their experience of success. This may be done directly, through group process, as well as through adapting the project to a family's level of ability.

In the free-play period, parents and children are afforded the opportunity to choose their own activity. The choices depend on the location of the group, the availability of games and equipment, and the ages of the children. Puzzles, table-top games, balls, gross motor games, dolls and materials for fantasy play may be available. The importance of this period of time is to promote negotiation and discussion among children and their parents about an activity that would be satisfying to both parties. In addition, parents learn more about their children's interests and learn how to adapt the games for their children's optimal engagement. Children also learn how to shift their own activity plans in order to engage their parents.

Leadership role

To develop a group environment that fosters positive interactions within families and among different families strong leadership skills are required. Leaders must provide a clear and organised group structure and implicit rules, so that they may focus on being a consultant to parents and simultaneously an advocate for children. To avoid having one's role limited to that of a supply provider, the group room should be set up and the range of potential activities for the entire group should be decided upon and organized by the leaders before the group begins and readily available during the group. Families are encouraged to get additional supplies that they may need during an activity and to clean up at the conclusion of the activity. The leaders should not be using their time to hunt for materials or to clean up after families. Therefore, the group room should be set up in a manner that allows this. In this way, families are empowered: they take on an active role as opposed to being guests and passive recipients. This also provides opportunities for interaction and negotiation between parent and child.

Before coming to the group, parents and children must understand the rules and structure of the group. An important rule is that each family engages in activity with one another. No family member is permitted to join another family. Two or more families may decide to play a large group game, but it must be negotiated within each family unit first and the activity must be appropriate for all family members. A game of basketball may be inappropriate for a 4-year-old child or for a mother in high heels.

In choosing activities for a parent–child activity group, occupational therapists analyse the interactional patterns between parent and child, and adapt the activity to increase the ability of both parent and child to participate successfully. This type of activity analysis is complex. Therapists need to examine activities from the perspective of both parent and child, as well as to consider how activities can facilitate the parent and child playing and working as collaboratively as possible. The role and dignity of parents as care-givers needs to be respected, while the developmental needs of children must also be considered.

Appropriate social behaviour is strongly encouraged throughout a parent–child activity group. No cursing, hitting, insulting or destruction of property is allowed. If parents do not set limits, the leaders address behaviour with children and invite parents to be a part of the discussion. Typically parents readily follow the lead of therapists. A leader states some appropriate responses to the misbehaviour that may be taken. Eye contact is made with the child, the parent and other group members. The goal is to avoid putting a parent on the spot, to give them a chance to absorb what has occurred, and to engage them in handling the situation effectively. If parents are unable or unwilling to engage in limit-setting with their children, then the leader carries out an intervention and serves as a role model. After the group, the leader should seek such parents to discuss the parents' perceptions of their children's behaviour and to the situation that occurred.

Leaders make parents feel competent by helping them to understand the project first and by helping them to cue their own children as opposed to watching a professional interact with their children. Guiding parents to experience success with their children will probably engage parents with their children and encourage future similar interactions. At the same time, leaders promote respect for children's feelings and autonomy, the use of kind but firm limits, positive reinforcement, the focus on the positive as opposed to the negative aspects of a project or interaction, and the expectation of improvement and cooperation. If children appear to be frustrated by their parents' inattention or over-involvement in a project, a leader may say: 'I bet if you told your mother that you were frustrated, I bet that she would be willing to help you'. Sometimes, this is all that is needed to cue a parent and redirect their attention toward their children. At other times, parents may express frustration back at their children; the leader then quietly helps a parent–child dyad to restructure the activity tasks so that both parties have a role that is satisfying to them. At times, parents have low frustration tolerance for their child's misbehaviour; they may threaten to leave if the child does not do exactly what they say. The leader might ask children to take a short time-out on a beanbag chair in the corner, allowing children, as well as their parents, to calm down so that they can re-engage in mutual activity after the time out. Making alternative suggestions and helping a family to carry out a reasonable plan that allows a parent and a child to calm down and then to re-approach the activity a short time later is enough to defuse a conflict that may have ended like many before them – with both parties becoming angry or hurt and deepening the rift between them. Parents have expressed gratitude with the assistance, and children have typically been responsive since their worst fears are often that their parents will actually leave and not come back.

Participant responses

When observing parents in a parent–child activity group, varied styles of coping with children's maladaptive behaviour can be seen. Some

---

Box 12.2 Case example: Ray

Ray was a 9-year-old boy with pervasive developmental disorder. His family was an intact middle-class family and both parents attended the group with him. Ray's mother was a teacher and his father was a postman. He had a 6-year-old sister who attended the group once Ray and his parents were consistently interacting successfully with group activities. Before hospitalization, Ray had been violent and aggressive at home.

In the initial group session that he attended, Ray exhibited significant problems in modulating his affect. He would become very excited if he liked an idea and would also become very angry when an idea did not work as he hoped it would. He was easily overstimulated, and became tense and anxious with any task or interpersonal challenge. His parents tried to interject ideas to help him as he tried to construct, but they presented their ideas in a way that was confusing to Ray. He responded by rudely rejecting their help, but then could not resolve challenges in the activities on his own; his tenseness escalated. He, at times, crushed supplies, attempted to destroy part of his project or stormed away from the table to a beanbag chair in the corner. His parents attempted to set limits which Ray ignored, and they gave up helplessly.

The activity group process was a very important part of the intervention. All other families were working on their own projects, so the group atmosphere fostered Ray's and his parents' expectation that they should get back to work after Ray calmed down. Their activity interaction was structured by a leader. The parents were motivated and invested in trying to work with Ray, but had had very limited success in the past and did not have any alternative strategies than the ones that they had unsuccessfully used in the past. A leader helped Ray's parents to break down the steps for projects that they could then offer a step-by-step plan to Ray. They were helped to limit the stimulation of additional supplies around their child. Along with the leader, the parents discussed with Ray that his goal for participating in the group was to allow them to help him and to work on a family project. As their help was now more organizing for Ray, he gradually accepted it, collaborated with them on his terms in completing a family project, and exhibited pleasure in his family's success in creating contraptions and constructions that they envisioned together.

After five sessions, the family began reporting to the group leaders that they had applied what they learned in group to family activities at home. They had successfully cleaned their hamster cages, prepared a family snack and played table-top games using some of the strategies that they were learning in the group.

---

parents appear to be walking on eggshells, afraid that their children might have a tantrum if they set limits. They seem to do whatever their children demand to get through the first groups that they attend. Other parents actively avoid interaction with their children in activity; they appear angry and ready for trouble between themselves and their children. Some parents take over projects from their children, who respond to the situation with the kind of misbehaviour that their parents seem to expect. As parents and children become comfortable in the group and began to use the support and assistance of the group leaders and other members, children remain more consistently involved in activity with their parents and the activities are more child directed. Children are reprimanded less, and parents and children exhibit more pleasure in their interaction. Over time, parents exhibit more interest in participating in activities with their children on and off the inpatient unit. Some also appear to develop a more optimistic view of interacting with their children. Parents report that their

initial pessimism about productively interacting with their children in group lessens. They report that watching other families participate in activities and listening to them discuss successes, as well as difficulties, were very helpful in changing their own expectations of their children. Other professionals have reported that, after participating in a parent–child activity group over a period of time, some parents and children are more positively engaged with one another at other times and more open to other forms of therapy.

Parents often express pleasant surprise in their children's ability to construct and to express pleasure in their work within a structured parent–child group. In the past, some parents reported that their children avoided these kinds of tasks or became easily angered when confronted by a challenge in the task. Having had this experience, parents begin to consider what adaptations their children need to participate successfully in constructional play. They also often bring up their concerns about how they might apply their group experiences to

Box 12.3 Case example: Valerie

Valerie was a 14-year-old girl who was psychiatrically hospitalized as a result of an episode of major depression and a suicide attempt. She also exhibited oppositional behaviour disorder and schizoid personality disorder. Valerie was one of four children who stated that she was never close to her siblings and had a tense relationship with her parents. She sat through family therapy sessions, but did not participate. Valerie and her mother, Mrs Smith, were referred to a parent–adolescent group. Mrs Smith was very talkative, but Valerie kept her physical distance from her mother and did not talk.

Valerie did talk to a leader before the group and planned to work on painting T-shirts, parallel to her mother. The activity facilitated interaction between mother and daughter. Valerie was very comfortable with the task; her mother was not. Valerie was encouraged to assist her mother, which Mrs Smith readily accepted. They then interacted comfortably around the activity. At the end of the activity, Valerie asked her mother to visit with her on the unit; she had not previously invited her mother to visit. The following week, Valerie planned a cooking activity with her mother. This was less successful because her mother had more skill; Valerie followed her mother's directions but was verbally hostile at times and physically and emotionally distant. The activity limited the autonomy that Valerie seemed to need to experience with her mother.

In the following weeks, Valerie was encouraged to plan painting or constructional tasks since she was more relaxed, animated and engaged while participating in these projects, and more skilled than her mother in them as well. Valerie and her mother needed the support and assistance of a group leader to begin such projects, but, once engaged, Valerie willingly helped her mother and then began to collaborate with her on constructions such a large papier mâché person. Valerie took the lead and her mother followed. Valerie enjoyed this and became more open to conversation about everyday things with her mother as they worked. With control in the activity, Valerie began to express more warmth towards her mother, and Mrs Smith noted strengths in her adolescent daughter of which she had not been aware previously. As she experienced pleasure in interacting with her mother in the parent–adolescent group, Valerie began participating in family therapy sessions and in activity with her mother outside of the hospital.

structuring play with their children at home (see Boxes 12.2 & 12.3). This provides the leaders with a window to assist families in generalising their group experiences. It can also lead to families problem-solving with each other and offering one another viable suggestions. This, of course, is very empowering and supports hope for the future which these families need.

PEER INTERACTION

Peer group work is central to the practice of occupational therapy within child psychiatry. To participate fully in childhood activities, children must have the sufficient interpersonal, play and task skills to be members of many formal and informal groups. Children are asked to be members of peer groups in school, after-school and community activities, as well as in informal groups that regularly develop among children on a playground or in a neighbourhood. To be accepted by peers, children need to invite and engage with other children in play, follow the rules of games and activities, be able to share and negotiate with peers, offer compliments and kind words to peers, help and accept

help from others. Children with mental illness often lack these basic social skills (Fig. 12.2).

To engage elementary school-aged children with mental illness in therapeutic group activities, Florey & Greene (1997) model their group work on the typical club activities of childhood that are very attractive to this age group. For example, they advocate running a boys' or a girls' scouting club that follows the structure of a typical girl or boy scout troop. Children design

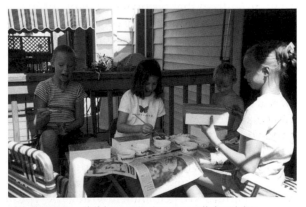

Figure 12.2 Children enjoying a parallel activity.

special club T-shirts and don them over their clothes at the start of group meetings. They may also create and use special signs or handshakes to greet members and to begin meetings. The group sequence follows the typical sequence of clubs. There are club rules that are drawn up by members and posted for all to refer to. Minutes of meetings are kept, and the minutes of the last meeting are read before beginning a new club activity. Florey & Greene's work highlights rituals and depersonalized controls, which are two critical elements that are emphasised in the psychodynamic literature about children's groups. Rituals can be organizing and comforting for all persons; they allow a person to anticipate what is to come and reinforce the connections among people who share the rituals. Depersonalised controls refer to rules and limits that are inherent in an activity and that come from the needs of a group and its activity. They are not rules developed by an authority figure or directed at any person; the rules arise from the group activity.

Olson (1999) addresses the need of some children with psychiatric disorders to develop sufficient play skills to participate in the group play occupations of childhood. If a child is not competent in activities in which peers are typically engaged, the child will probably experience rejection from the other children. Within a therapeutic activity group, children can be provided with the opportunity to build basic play and task skills, as they develop social skills.

It may also be important to consider what emotional needs certain play and leisure occupations may provide so that occupations may optimally meet children's emotional needs. Caring for pets versus playing a sport or a competitive game meets different needs relative to emotional development. Children may not explore a broad range of activities that could potentially meet their needs because of underlying sensorimotor, cognitive, coping or social skills, or an insufficient opportunity. Therapists need to foster exploration of varied activities that may foster psychological, cognitive and physical development. Olson (1997) discusses the potential psychological benefits of participation in a range of typical childhood activities.

Dealing with bias and the 'isms': racism, sexism

In a multicultural society such as the United States, it is not surprising that racism, bias or prejudice affect the dynamics of many groups in which people from different cultures interact. Although there have been many changes within the legal and educational system in the United States to foster equality among people of different races and cultures, and to support women in education and the workforce, racism and sexism are still part of the everyday experiences of persons of colour, women and homosexuals. Some talk disparagingly about women or people who belong to minorities in everyday conversation; most do not. It is generally considered impolite and ignorant to talk in this way. Many white Americans believe that racism is a problem of the past that has been successfully abolished. But jokes with persons who are not male, white or heterosexual as the foil are commonplace and at times ignored even by members of minorities. Although there have been important gains in the presentation of women and minorities in the media, the media continue to support the white middle class culture as the ideal and other cultures as inferior. The young African American male who wanders into a white neighbourhood is seen as a potential criminal by many passers by.

Sometimes an occupational therapy student will ask: 'What do the larger societal issues have to do with therapeutic group work with children and adolescents? In these groups, everyone gets along. The problems that occur between members are just related to the children's mental illness'. In my experience, as well as in the reports of my occupational therapy students, prejudicial comments are common in group interaction. Over the past few years, I have studied the experiences of my students as they co-led groups for children and adolescents with mental illness.

Prejudicial comments may go unnoticed or ignored as background noise, but they influence group dynamics in subtle (although sometimes blatant) ways. They limit the therapeutic impact of groups. It may be painful to believe that children could exhibit prejudice or racist behaviour or that a leader's own unexamined biases might reflect a deep problem for the healthy functioning of a group. What follows are some vignettes from my students' logs to illustrate some of the issues that may surface within a group.

One student who was in her early twenties wrote:

Although I know that race can play a major role in group dynamics. I find that I do not like to look for racial problems. I prefer to give people the benefit of the doubt that they are fair and open-minded – especially younger generations who have been raised with more understanding of the importance of equal rights and impartial treatment.

A few weeks later, she wrote:

I received a wake-up call following a group session 2 weeks ago. My co-leader and I were trying to explain to a group member that we would not be able to go fishing as a group. Sam started to say something, but stifled himself, stating that he couldn't say it because it was racial. He then whispered the comment in my co-leader's ear. She told me that he said, 'I don't want to do nigger activities'. My co-leader responded, 'We didn't today, did we?' I continue to wonder what a nigger activity is in Sam's eyes.

Sometimes the tables are turned: in some residential settings, the majority of the children are from minority backgrounds. In one group, a child of Jamaican heritage stated: 'I don't want to work with these stupid white folk'.

Sociocultural issues often remain unaddressed until there is a major conflict, sometimes including physical violence. One student wrote about an altercation between two adolescents:

Mark and Lee had been arguing about the television set. When Mark was leaving the room and bumped into Lee's foot, Lee took it as an affront. He called Mark a 'dumb Iranian' and an 'Arab' and said that he was 'sick and tired of living with a dumb Iranian Arab'. Mark defended himself by saying, 'I was born here, my father is Iranian and I'm American!'. Lee and Mark cursed at each other and then Lee punched Mark in the face. The two were told that they had one night to resolve their differences or there would be a room change. The conflict was not resolved and the result was a room and floor change for Mark. Mark was happy to move; he said that Lee gave him too much stress.

Sometimes the leader is the target of bias; one student wrote:

Most of the children asked me if I was Chinese. Before I could answer, the children started to call out 'chink-chonk'. One of the group members said that all Chinese people have flat faces and noses and that I am so ugly. Some of the children squinted their eyes and slanted their eyes with their hands. It was like a domino effect as one child led the giggling, followed by another and another. The echoes started throughout the room. I took this as the way that the children welcomed my presence.

The last sentence seems to highlight how a therapist may interpret bias or racism exhibited in a group as meaning something other than bias or racism. It may feel too uncomfortable to address as it may be in reality. The same Asian American student wrote:

I was very shocked at the comments made by the group members. It was hard to believe that such young children are aware of racial issues. I avoided the situation and hope that I will be able to gain their trust before I can talk about the racial issues that they have with me. My readings suggest that a therapist should discuss race and racial issues, but I am reluctant to do so. I have often used the avoidance response when I encountered racism and prejudice. I do not like to have confrontations with anybody, but I have felt angry and hostile at times.

It was important for this student to reflect on her own feelings and to find a way openly to discuss racial differences within her group for her own competence as a therapist and for the emotional and social growth of the children in her group. It is likely that the children in her group have experienced similar reactions from other children or from adults in response to their minority status in the United States. Having the opportunity to observe an adult deal with bias openly and effectively may change children's thinking and lead to more open and productive discussion of issues related to racism.

About an interaction in another group, a student wrote:

Tommy was awarded the Resident of the Week. His prize was a McDonald's Happy Meal. Tanya noticed that Tommy was sharing his soda with his brother and another boy at their table. Tanya asked if she could have some soda also. Tommy replied, 'No! Only white people can have some. I don't want your germs.'

Although children are not typically seen as being capable of exhibiting prejudicial or racist

become easily frustrated in play. They never seem to 'get it right', no matter how hard they try. It is not a matter of insufficient effort or practice in activities, but a matter of deficient development of their underlying capacities.

When addressing this area of dysfunction in treatment, therapists typically use a range of suspended swings and related equipment to provide children with sufficiently intense and organised vestibular, tactile and proprioceptive input. In this way, an optimal alert state, improved muscle tone, postural stability and endurance are facilitated so that children are physically ready to participate in sensorimotor play that will support their development of eye–hand and bilateral motor coordination. Different swings foster development of flexion and extension, and put different demands on children's postural control and balance. Riding a net swing may be used to foster extension against gravity and provide strong input leading to increased stability of the upper extremities. A pony swing can be used to foster whole-body flexion and to foster balance reactions. While children ride on equipment, therapists foster play so that children incorporate their developing support capabilities naturally into their everyday occupation – play. As children swing prone in a net swing, they may play target games or retrieve letters to play word games (Fig.

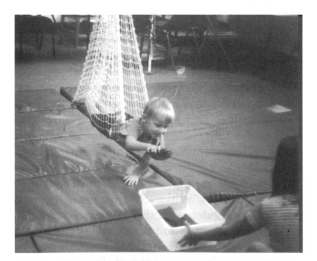

Figure 12.4 A child throwing bean bags into a box as he swings.

12.4). With an appropriate level of challenge, children's behaviour will be organised and they will be alert and focused, and ready to develop new skills. If children begin to be more engaged and invested in play within therapy, they will likely seek out similar experiences within therapy and within secure situations outside therapy.

Praxis

Besides developing their sensory processing skills and underlying support capacities, children must also develop their praxis abilities in order to succeed in their everyday occupations. They need to generalize what they have learned in other activities to new activities with which they are confronted and to plan out an approach to a new piece of equipment or activity based upon their previous experiences with other activities. Many children with underlying sensory processing disorders exhibit deficits related to praxis.

Within therapy, children are regularly confronted with novel equipment or new challenges with familiar equipment. They may be asked to think of a new way to ride a swing or to help the therapist figure out a 'fun' way to play with a new piece of equipment. As children explore equipment in novel ways, they build up motor memories, explore their own body scheme, and learn to plan new motor tasks. It is then easier for them to explore and master everyday play occupations such as skipping rope which is a demanding motor task to learn.

To learn more about sensory integration and the typical methods of assessment and treatment used by therapists trained in this frame of reference, it is suggested that readers first read Kranowitz's (1998) book *The Out of Synch Child*, which is an easy-to-read introduction to sensory integration written for parents and professionals alike. For more in-depth coverage, Kimball's chapters in *Frames of Reference for Pediatric Occupational Therapy* (Kimball 1999a, b) provide a concise, clear overview and description of how to use the sensory integration frame of reference.

Incorporating Greenspan's approach to emotional development with sensory integration

Many therapists in the United States have embraced the work of Stanley Greenspan, a well known child psychiatrist. They use his methods conjointly with sensory integration methods to engage young children with regulatory or multi-system developmental disorders. These diagnoses are part of the *Diagnostic Classification of Mental Health and Developmental Disorders of Infancy and Early Childhood* (1994), which was developed by a task force of Zero to Three/National Center for Clinical Infant Programs, chaired by Greenspan. These diagnoses acknowledge the role that sensory processing and sensorimotor development play in the mental health and developmental functioning of young children. Children with regulatory disorders exhibit behavioural difficulties, which may include behavioural control or social difficulties in addition to difficulties regulating physiological, sensory, motor and affective states. Children with multisystem developmental disorder exhibit significant disorders in communication, motor and sensory processing, but reveal a greater capacity or potential for intimacy and closeness than do children with autism. Occupational therapy services that emphasise sensory integration treatment methods are typically recommended for children with these disorders.

Greenspan has developed a framework for understanding the development of personality in young children. His model attempts to explain how constitutional–maturational and interactional factors affect the way in which children move through emotional developmental levels. The constitutional–maturational factors include sensory processing and reactivity, motor tone and motor planning. Greenspan works closely with occupational therapists to address these factors. Interactional factors simply refer to the manner in which parents and other care-givers engage with children.

Constitutional factors may hinder children's availability for interaction. Children who are hypersensitive to sensory input may withdraw from physical contact and social engagement, which will interfere with their emotional growth. Parents may attempt to engage children at the particular children's emotional developmental level or they may approach children as much younger or older children. The latter may limit emotional growth.

The stages of emotional development that Greenspan (1997) has identified are:

1. Shared attention and engagement. This develops in the first months of life and refers to children learning to look, listen to and attend to care-givers.
2. Two way communication. This milestone begins as simple gestural communication between parent and child, and leads to more complex communication patterns that include words and gestures.
3. Shared meanings. Play at this level involves expressions of emotion; pretend play is typical of this stage.
4. Emotional thinking. At this level, children categorise emotions and make connections between emotion and behaviour.

Greenspan teaches parents and other professionals to consider at what developmental level specific children are presently functioning and to engage the child at that particular level. He fosters a reflective style in care-givers, who watch children's spontaneous play and then find a way to communicate with children within their play. His method of facilitating children's emotional development includes a process called 'Floortime'. This is a period of play between a child and a care-giver during which the care-giver follows the lead of the child and works to open and close circles of communication.

A circle of communication is opened when an individual does or says something that another person can imitate or expand upon. A circle is closed when another individual says or does something in response to the play action of the first person. A child may roll a toy car across the room; a therapist closes the circle of communication by intercepting it. The child may then open another circle of communication to let the care-giver know that he or she did not like what the care-giver did or to incorporate the care-giver's action into the play. The care-giver closes each circle of communication with another response which encourages the child to open another circle of communication. The goals of the care-giver are to engage children on their terms and to extend the number and complexity of circles of communication. In this way, more mature and elaborate social play develops. Through consistent and regular experiences in Floortime with care-givers, children develop the capacity to share meanings with others in play and to attach emotional meanings in play. To learn more about Floortime, Greenspan (1992) and the video 'Understanding Children's Emotions' (Benham 1990) are recommended.

Therapists apply Greenspan's concepts of Floortime in activities they use to engage children in a therapy session. As occupational therapists foster improved sensory modulation and integration, they also may foster children's emotional development and capacity for social play.

SUMMARY

Although few occupational therapists in the United States work with children and adolescents with psychiatric disorders, occupational therapists who work with this population have developed dynamic intervention strategies to foster occupational development and performance. Peer and family group occupations have been a focus in the literature that has been produced. Therapists also address coping and sensory processing capacities in some children and adolescents, as dysfunction in these underlying performance components may be significant barriers to psychosocial health.

REFERENCES

Ainsworth M 1967 Object relations, dependency and attachment: a theoretical review of the infant–mother relationship. Child Development 40:969–1020
American Occupational Therapy Association 1995 Position paper: occupation. American Journal of Occupational Therapy 49:1015–1018
Arend R, Gore R L, Sroufe L A 1979 Continuity of individual adaptation from infancy to kindergarten: a predictive

study of ego resilience and curiosity in preschoolers. Child Development 50:950–957
Ayres A J 1972 Sensory integration and learning disorder. Western Psychological Service, Los Angeles
Ayres A J 1989 Sensory integration and praxis tests. Western Psychological Service, Los Angeles
Benham H 1990 Understanding children's emotions. Early Childhood Division, Scholastic (video)
Coster W 1997 School function assessment. Therapy Skill Builders, San Antonio, Texas
Dunn W 1997a The impact of sensory processing abilities on the daily lives of young children and their families: a conceptual model. Infants and Young Children 48:967–974
Dunn W 1997b The sensory profile: a discriminating measure of sensory processing in daily life. Sensory Integration Special Interest Section Quarterly of the American Occupational Therapy Association 20(1):1–3
Dunn W, Westman K 1997 The sensory profile: the performance of a national sample of children without disabilities. American Journal of Occupational Therapy 51:25–34
Fidler G S, Fidler J W 1978 Doing and becoming: purposeful action and self-actualization. American Journal of Occupational Therapy 32:305–310
Fisher A G 1998 Uniting practice and theory in an occupational framework: 1998 Eleanor Clarke Slagle lecture. American Journal of Occupational Therapy 52:509–521
Fisher A G, Murray E A, Bundy A C 1991 Sensory integration: theory and practice. F A Davis, Philadelphia
Florey L L, Greene S 1997 Play in middle childhood: a focus on children with behavior and emotional disorders. In: Parham L D, Faxio L S (eds) Play in occupational therapy for children. Mosby, St Louis, p 126
Greenberg M T, Speltz M L, DeKlyen M 1993 The role of attachment in the early development of disruptive behavior problems. Development and Psychopathology 5:191–213
Greenspan S I 1992 Infancy and early childhood – the practice of clinical assessment and intervention with emotional and developmental challenges. International Universities Press, Madison, Connecticut
Greenspan S 1997 The developmental structuralist model of early personality development. In: Noshpitz J, Greenspan S, Wieder S, Osofsky J (eds) Handbook of child and adolescent psychiatry, vol 1: infants and preschoolers. John Wiley, New York, p 351
Heard D H 1981 From object relations to attachment theory: a basis for family therapy. British Journal of Medical Psychology 51:67–76
Kimball J G 1999a Sensory integration frame of reference: theoretical base, function/dysfunction continua, and guide to evaluation. In: Kramer P, Hinojosa J (eds) Frames of reference for pediatric occupational therapy, 2nd edn. Lippincott Williams & Wilkins, Baltimore, p 119
Kimball J G 1999b Sensory integration frame of reference: postulates regarding change and application to practice. In: Kramer P, Hinojosa J (eds) Frames of reference for pediatric occupational therapy, 2nd edn. Lippincott Williams & Wilkins, Baltimore, p 169
Kranowitz C S 1998 The out of synch child: recognizing and coping with sensory integration dysfunction. Skylight Press: New York
Moyers P A 1999 The guide to occupational therapy practice. American Journal of Occupational Therapy 53:247–322

Murphy L 1962 The widening world of childhood. Basic Books, New York.

Murphy L, Moriarty A 1976 Vulnerability, coping and growth: from infancy to adolescence. Yale University Press, New Haven, Connecticut.

Olson L J 1997 Sublimations of the grade school child. In: Noshpitz J D, Kernberg P, Bemporad J (eds) Handbook of child and adolescent psychiatry, vol 2. John Wiley, New York, p 107

Olson L J 1999 Psychosocial frame of reference. In: Kramer P, Hinojosa J (eds) Frames of reference for pediatric occupational therapy, 2nd edn. Lippincott Williams & Wilkins, Baltimore, p 323

Olson L, Heaney C, Soppas-Hoffman B 1989 Parent–child activity group treatment in preventive psychiatry. Occupational Therapy in Health Care 6(1):29 43

Reilly M (ed) 1974 Play as exploratory learning. Sage, Beverly Hills

Schultz S 1992 School-based occupational therapy for students with behavioral disorders. Occupational Therapy in Health Care 8:173–196

Sue D W, Sue D 1990 Counseling the culturally different: theory and practice, 2nd edn. John Wiley, New York

Sylva K 1984 A hard-headed look at the fruits of play. Early Child Development and Care 15:171–184

Takata N 1974 Play as a prescription. In: Reilly M (ed) Play as exploratory learning. Sage, Thousand Oaks, California, p 209

Tatum B T 1997 Why are all the black kids sitting together in the cafeteria? and other conversations about race. Basic Books, New York

Trombly C A 1995 Occupation: purposefulness and meaningfulness as therapeutic mechanisms: 1995 Eleanor Clarke Slagle lecture. American Journal of Occupational Therapy 49:960–972

Waters E, Wittman J, Sroufe L A 1979 Attachment, positive affect and competence in the peer group: two studies in construct validation. Child Development 50:821–829

Wilbarger P 1991 Sensory defensiveness in children aged 2–12 (Booklet). Avanti Educational Programs, Denver, Colorado.

Wilbarger P 1995 The sensory diet: activity programs based on sensory processing theory. Sensory Integration Special Interest Section Quarterly of the American Occupational Therapy Association 18(2):1–4

Williams M S, Shellenberger S 1994 How does your engine run? A leader's guide to the alert program for self regulation. Therapyworks, Albuquerque, New Mexico

Williamson G G, Szczepanski M 1999 Coping frame of reference. In: Kramer P, Hinojosa J (eds) Frames of reference for pediatric occupational therapy, 2nd edn. Lippincott Williams & Wilkins, Baltimore, p 431

Wood W 1995 Weaving the warp and weft of occupational therapy: an art and science for all times. American Journal of Occupational Therapy 49:44–52

Yalom I 1975 The theory and practice of group psychotherapy. Basic Books, New York

Zeitlin S 1985 Coping inventory: a measure of adaptive behavior. Scholastic Testing Service, Bensenville, Illinois

Zero to Three 1994 Diagnostic classification of mental health and developmental disorders of infancy and early childhood. National Center for Clinical Infant Programs, Arlington, Virginia

13

Child, adolescent and family occupational therapy services in New Zealand

Ann Christie   Rowena Scaletti

INTRODUCTION

New Zealand is a small country in the South Pacific with a population of 3.8 million people. It is multicultural, the indigenous Maori people having been joined over time by immigrants from Europe, Asia and Pacific Islands. The Treaty of Waitangi, signed in 1840, is the partnership document between Maori and the State, and is considered the beginning of New Zealand's nationhood (Tauroa 1989). It is the foundation of services to all New Zealanders, including health. In return for Maori conceding sovereign rights to the British Crown, they were guaranteed that the Crown would actively protect Maori tribal authority over their lands, fisheries, forests and culture. The Crown also extended to Maori the status and rights of British citizens (Project Waitangi 1992). Implicit in the Treaty are concepts of equity, partnership, and economic and cultural security, all of which contribute to hauora or the spirit of life and health.

The New Zealand health system has seen over a decade of health service reform (Mooney & Salmond 1994) and a division between service funder (central government through Transitional Health Authorities and the Central Funding Authority) and providers (public, private and non-profit hospitals and other organisations). Following the change of government in 1999 it is intended to dissolve the funder/provider split. District Health Boards (DHB) will be developed, each responsible for 'deciding the mix, level and quality of health and disability services' (King 2000, p. 1). DHBs will be clearly and formally accountable to the Minister of Health.

Funding for health care derives mainly from general taxation (Scott 1994), changes to health provision being driven by public sector cost containment. Funding may be provided on a permanent basis as in funding public hospital-based child and adolescent mental health services and community agencies, or as limited interventions to target specific areas of need, for example adolescent suicide or child sexual abuse. These are reviewed and renewed, or not, depending on outcomes.

Children and adolescents account for approximately 23% of the New Zealand population, yet over the years mental health services have received relatively little attention or funding (McGeorge 1995). Conservative estimations suggest that in New Zealand 5% of children and adolescents have a serious psychiatric disorder that requires specialist intervention (Mason 1996). It was estimated only 1% of this population were receiving treatment from specialist services (McGeorge 1995).

Additional funding has been made available more recently as an outcome of the 1996 Mason Inquiry into the effectiveness and efficiency of mental health treatment in New Zealand. This has released extra funding for child and adolescent mental health services, identified as priority areas of need. In addition, some non-government agencies gain funding from Trusts, local government, banks, businesses, churches and fee-paying clients on a sliding scale commensurate with income.

Alternative funding is also available through central government for specific initiatives in mental health. One such initiative is funding for those affected by domestic violence through the enactment in 1995 of the Domestic Violence Act. Individual and group therapy programmes are now available for protected persons as well as offenders. Programmes may be approved for up to 2 years, at which time providers must reapply for funding approval.

A review of progress since 1995 (Mental Health Commission 1999) shows an increase in community-based child and youth mental health services through the expansion of existing services and the development of new services. Based on the benchmarks identified in the Blueprint for Mental Health Services (Mental Health Commission 1998) this expansion is planned through to 2002 (Health Funding Authority 1998).

It is hoped that a Chair of Child and Adolescent Psychiatry (child and adolescent mental health) will be established in the future at the Auckland University School of Medicine (Mental Health Commission 1999). It is intended to appoint a professor to lead a teaching and research unit. It is acknowledged that the major contributing factors in the development of mental health disorders appear to be the lack of self-esteem, depression, lack of access to professionals, and inadequate support services for clients. This is seen as balancing the commitment between adult and child services.

The impact of changes in the health sector on occupational therapy services in New Zealand has not been extensively researched. Thomas (1994) acknowledged that enforced change was difficult for everyone within the health services, and Fechner (1991) and Kendall (1994) focused on the need for strong, professional leadership, professional mentors and knowledge. The impact of change in the health sector on the feelings of satisfaction and frustration of occupational therapists working with children and families was researched in 1997 (Scaletti 1997), and it appears occupational therapists are adapting to changing demands – albeit with some stress – on their professional services.

The changing New Zealand health system, together with increasing focus on financial and professional accountability, provides impetus for the continuing redefinition of the occupational therapy role in child and adolescent mental health. Over the past 18 years three occupational therapists, Manley, Scaletti and Christie, have largely influenced role development. Working over time within the Auckland Child and Family Unit as part of a multidisciplinary team they have made their own unique and significant contributions to the face of occupational therapy (Scaletti & Christie 1996, Christie 1999b). Traditional paediatric occupational therapy, with emphasis on child development and role acquisition, and later sensory integration procedures, were the initial focus. To establish credibility within the team, research projects (Christie & Robertson 1991, 1993, Werry, Scaletti & Mills 1990) and collaboration with team members were used to support and develop the occupational therapy service. As traditional occupational therapy services moved into the community, occupational therapists in child and family units have responded to the need to become more consultative in their practice.

There are fewer positions for occupational therapists in child and adolescent mental health outside the Auckland area. The Christchurch Child and Family Mental Health Service offers both regional inpatient and outpatient facilities for children and adolescents. It employs one occupational therapist, who assesses and treats patients with a range of diagnoses. Traditional occupational therapy theories, models and frames of references, such as the Model of Human Occupation (Keilhofner 1992), sensory integration (Fisher, Murray & Bundy 1991) and neurodevelopmental (Shoen & Anderson 1993), inform this role. The newly established adolescent day programme employs four staff, one of whom is an occupational therapist.

As more students are graduating with field work experience in child and adolescent mental health increased opportunities are being developed for occupational therapists. Local resources, strong supervision, and telecommunication support them with Auckland occupational therapists assisting them in their role development.

Two Schools of Occupational Therapy in New Zealand offer Bachelor degree-level courses, with one also offering a postgraduate diploma. Masters' degrees in occupational therapy are taught in conjunction with the University of South Australia, or may be taken through long-distance study directly from Australia. The degree of Doctor of Philosophy is also available through long distance study from Australia. Occupational therapists are also able to participate in generic Masters and PhD programmes from a variety of tertiary institutions across New Zealand. In 2000 there were 2257 registered occupational therapists in New Zealand (Occupational Therapy Board Newsletter 2000), most working in the public health service. In total there are approximately 16 occupational therapists working in child and mental health in New Zealand, 10 in Auckland and six elsewhere.

Occupational therapists are acutely aware of the need to work with individuals and families within their own cultural values. Frequently, workers are employed primarily for their cultural knowledge – an acknowledgment of the essential nature of cultural traditions and beliefs in the healing process. As Durie, writing about New Zealand mental health in 1984 stated, 'the notions of mental health are bound by culture and time, and thus mental health cannot be isolated from whanau (extended family), culture, spirituality, and the environment' (p. 5). That is, the concept of 'mental health' depends on cultural values and beliefs of the time (Ivey, Ivey & Simek-Morgan 1993).

A longitudinal study (Whitehead 1995) concerning occupational therapy students' perceptions of cultural difference is presently being undertaken in New Zealand in conjunction with the University of British Colombia, Canada. The findings at this stage of the study indicate that 'students' perceptions of themselves as people influenced their perceptions of cultural difference' (p. 291).

Multiskilling has also become an essential element for New Zealand occupational therapists to contend with. Although 'every profession has core constructs . . . through which it obtains identity' (Hodgson 1992, p. 45), many health services in New Zealand employ on the basis of skill, not profession. Frequently, occupational therapists are now seen as working 'generically', part of a group of people with common characteristics (Collins Dictionary 1990). Through necessity, occupational therapists are up-skilling, building on existing skills and developing additional skills. It has become essential that, for occupational therapy to present as a profession that can continue to adapt to changes in the health sector, formal education, workshops, training courses and external supervision become part of every occupational therapist's professional climate.

The New Zealand Association of Occupational Therapists (NZAOT) (1998, p. 16) acknowledges that the following values guide the work of the New Zealand Association of Occupational Therapists.

The New Zealand Association of Occupational Therapists:

- values the partnership inherent in the Treaty of Waitangi
- believes all New Zealanders have the right to equitable access to healthcare and the support they need
- believes all New Zealanders have the right to access occupational therapy services they need
- values the importance of each individual and their family/whanau and wider community, and believes that each person has the right to be an active participant

- values diversity and believes that all people, of whatever age, gender, ethnic origin, culture, sexual orientation, or ability are valuable members of the community
- believes that every person has the right to be involved in occupations that have meaning and purpose for them, and that this is vital for them to maintain wellness
- believes that all people have the right to dignity, privacy, respect, and to appropriate levels of information, choice and autonomy
- values relationships based on partnership and mutual respect
- values the guidance of consumers regarding effective service delivery
- values its members, and encourages their feedback and active participation
- believes that a collective voice for occupational therapists is important
- places a high value on quality, and believes that a quality service requires a competent and skilled workforce
- values accountability, ethical practice, high professional standards of practice, commitment to continuing professional development
- values the ongoing advancement of occupational knowledge and skills through research.

This chapter describes the clinical practice of occupational therapists working in child and adolescent mental health: a central government-funded community child, adolescent and family service, and a community child and family service in the not-for-profit sector (non-government organisation). An overview of models of practice used in clinical practice is shown in Box 13.1.

AUCKLAND CHILD, ADOLESCENT AND FAMILY SERVICE: A STATE HEALTH SERVICE

Ann Christie

The Child and Family Unit (CFU) opened in Auckland in the early 1970s. It included inpatient, day-patient and outpatient facilities,

Box 13.1 Occupational therapy theories, models of practice, and frames of reference combined with treatment approaches that are used in New Zealand Child Mental Health Services

Main treatment approaches
Usually referred to as types of intervention towards problems or for role of the child.

- Directive and non-directive play – indoors and outdoors
- Family therapy
- Sensory integration procedures
- Cognitive-behavioural therapy
- Child developmental assessment and intervention
- Groups for children and adults
- Individual therapy for adults and children
- Creative and psychodynamic techniques
- Couple therapy – provided by some services

Models and theories

- Acquisitional theories — Rogers, Skinner, Bandura, Newell, Simon
- Adaptive skills — Cronin
- Canadian Model of Occupational Performance — Townsend et al
- Canadian Model of Social Competence — Doble & McGill
- Creative Problem Solving Model — Lewin & Reed
- Developmental theories — Freud, Erickson, Piaget, Kohlberg, Gesell, Maslow, Havighurst
- Family-centred approach — Case-Smith, Pratt & Allen
- Family therapy — Barker, Epston & White, Hayes, McKinnon & James
- Group models — Sattler, Corey
- Model of Human Occupation — Kielhofner
- Occupational behavioural approach — Matsutsuyu
- Operational theories: social learning, behaviour, psychosocial, emotional attachment — Bowlby, Chess & Thomas, Greenspan, Reilly
- Play theories — Reilly, Bundy, Florey, Morrison, Metzger, Pratt
- Play in occupational therapy — Bundy, Parham, Fazio
- Psychosocial components of occupational therapy — Mosey
- Psychodynamic theories — Corey
- Sensory integrative procedures — Ayres, Murray, Fisher, Bundy

Frames of reference

- Activities of daily living — Christiansen
- Analytical — Mosey, Bruce & Borg, Reed
- Behavioural — Bruce & Borg, Beck, Dryden
- Cognitive-behavioural — Bruce & Borg
- Coping — Williamson, Szczepanski & Zeitlin
- Developmental — Llorens
- Group work applied — Mosey, Kielhofner, Hopkins & Smith
- Holistic — Bruce & Borg
- Human occupation — O'Brien
- Neurodevelopmental — Shoen & Anderson
- Occupational behaviour — Reilly
- Psychosocial — Olsen
- Sensory integration — Kimball
- Spatiotemporal adaptation — Gilfoyle, Grady & Moore

and a schoolroom. An occupational therapist was employed part-time and worked autonomously within the team to provide both consultative and clinical occupational therapy practices. No treatment facilities were provided on-site: treatment facilities in the main occupational therapy department were used.

Traditionally the CFU supports one of the longest operating child mental health services, and has consistently employed occupational therapists. This was due, in part, to the support and encouragement of one of the consultant child psychiatrists, Professor John Werry, who recognised the value of occupational therapy and the diligence of the therapists employed in promoting their profession. The role of occupational therapy has continued to evolve with subsequent therapists contributing their specific skills and interpretation of what occupational therapy has to offer children with mental health problems.

In 1991 the CFU became part of the Starship Children's Hospital. Then, in 1996, as a result of a pilot study on the value of community-based services that involved the occupational therapist, the outpatient section of the CFU moved to the community to become Community Child, Adolescent and Family Service (CCAFS). In 1999 there were five full-time positions for occupational therapy in this service.

THE COMMUNITY CHILD, ADOLESCENT AND FAMILY SERVICE (CCAFS)

CCAFS, based within the community, is a service linked with the Starship Children's Hospital. It has four interrelated services and 55 full time equivalent staff.

Location

Located near the Starship Children's Hospital and the city centre, this catchment area, with a population of 345 750 and approximately 93 186 children within our age group (Walker 1996), covers a wide socioeconomic range of people and the main business area of Auckland.

Types of disorder

Typical problems fall into the categories of serious or suspected serious mental health issues, such as the DSM-IV (American Psychiatric Association 1994) criteria of severe emotional and behavioural disturbances, parenting problems, family conflict and eating disorders. Clients must be aged 17 years or less. Clients with abuse issues, drugs and alcohol, and family violence are seen by other local services.

Referrals

Clients reflect the DSM-IV criteria. Therapists are encouraged to develop skills in areas or disorders of interest, where occupational therapy models of practice offer children and their families opportunities for change, for example behavioural, anxiety and mood disorders, and other client types such as those with personality disorders, pervasive developmental disorders, depression and those in the refugee population (Lewis 1996, Rutter, Taylor & Hersov 1996). CCAFS cultural philosophy guides therapists to address the needs of our indigenous population (Fernando 1991) and an increasingly multicultural society (Holman 1994). Cultural advisers, working alongside clinicians, support Maori and Pacific Island peoples. Liaising with appropriate services supports other cultures.

Occupational therapists choose their caseload from the CCAFS allocation, interview and review processes, or following consultation with team members. Referrals are reliant on the therapist's ability to promote his or her role, relate theory to practice, and show effective clinical reasoning and reflective practice.

The CCAFS criteria for intervention must be met. Before being accepted for assessment and intervention, the client must have an identified child mental health issue. Children who present with activities of daily living (ADL), sensorimotor, sensory integration, learning or physical difficulties are referred to another community service. A further service, the James Family Centre, deals with child behaviour and parenting issues. In cases where the child presents with both mental health and physical problems, the intervention is shared

...es. In addition, where children ...ent with multiagency involve- ... is called for all professionals and ...ominate a key agency to manage the ca... ...uss how best to meet the intervention objecti... Box 13.2 describes CCAFS occupational therapy intervention where another service is involved in providing intervention in the school.

The CCAFS team

CCAFS is a free, culturally sensitive mental health service for children, young people and their families of the culturally diverse central district of

---

Box 13.3 The multidisciplinary team

- Consultant child and adolescent psychiatrists
- Cultural advisers (Pacific Island, Maori)
- Clinical psychologists
- Occupational therapists
- Family therapists
- Art therapist
- Psychiatric and paediatric registrars
- Psychiatric nurse therapists
- Social workers
- Speech and language therapist
- Spiritual advisor

Auckland City. The multidisciplinary team consists of people with backgrounds in various professions relating to mental health (Box 13.3). The four interrelated teams within the service are the Community Service Team (CST), Child Adolescent Liaison Service (CLS), the Youth Early Intervention Service (YEIS) and the Youth Forensic Service (YFS). All interrelated CCAFS teams liaise with the Child and Family Unit (CFU) at Starship Children's Hospital, although more specifically the YEIS team (Box 13.4).

The two liaison functions include:

1. experiential outpatient training for medics on clinical placement in the CFU. They share casework with the CCAFS team, which includes occupational therapists as their trainers.
2. referrals from CCAFS of children or adolescents requiring short-term inpatient admission.

Main treatment approaches

Assessments focus on psychosocial, psychological, emotional and sensory development, using theories that consider innate temperament, attachment, peer interaction, play, ability to cope and environmental interaction, and the challenges these occupations present for children (Olson 1993, Williamson, Szczepanski & Zeitlin 1993). Assessment may take place on site, at school or in the home (Hinojosa & Kramer 1993, Muhlenhaupt 1993). Few assessments are designed by our profession specifically to

---

Box 13.2 Case example: James

A public health nurse who had observed unusual playground behaviours during a scheduled school visit referred James, a 7-year-old boy, to CCAFS. Initial interview and assessment procedures revealed encopresis, sensory problems, motor and language dyspraxia, social and emotional difficulties. James was diagnosed with Asperger's syndrome. In keeping with a family-centred approach, objectives were set that included both the parents and James. Referrals were made to Developmental Paediatrics at the Starship Hospital to address the encopresis; to the Child Development Service to address the motor and language problems; to Special Education Services to address the learning problems; and notification was made to James's school outlining his multifaceted problems. A meeting with the family and agency representatives took place at which CCAFS was identified as the key agency. The intervention objectives were outlined and coordinated with other agency plans.

Initially, both occupational therapists consulted together then liaised with James's school to set up joint classroom therapy programmes. These programmes were regularly upgraded and adapted as James progressed. The CCAFS occupational therapy programme included psychoeducation for the family, school and support staff on Asperger's syndrome, including the implications for James on his developing cognitive, social and psychological areas of function. Classroom adaptation included visual support strategies to improve learning and behaviour (Attwood 1997, Ulliana & Mitchell 1998). In addition, intervention addressed the psychosocial, emotional and temperamental difficulties affecting James's occupational performance such as relationships, social skills, and the environmental stressors in the playground and home. Individual and group intervention took place on site, at home and in school. Six months later a further family group conference took place to monitor the intervention progress across settings.

Box 13.4 Interrelated CCAFS teams and CFU

Child and Adolescent Liaison Service (CLS)

This inter-related team is a specialist service devised to work with the social workers at the Department of Child, Youth and Family Service (CYFS) in the regional area of Auckland City. A consultation model of practice is used providing assessment, consultation, training and education in mental health issues for social workers. Identified clients are up to the age of 17 years and must have involvement with the associated CYFS. There are four multidisciplinary professionals on this team who consult when necessary with the CCAFS occupational therapist.

Youth Early Intervention Service (YEIS) (see Box 13.8)

This inter-related team provides a specialist service for children and adolescents (10–17 years) experiencing first episode psychosis, a screening process for those at risk of developing a psychosis, those recovering from a psychotic episode and severe anxiety disorders, i.e. obsessive–compulsive disorder (OCD). Through negotiation older adolescents may be seen providing they meet the criteria. The YEIS is also involved in working with schools and other agencies to promote an understanding of mental health difficulties and young people. This team has eight multidisciplinary professionals that include an occupational therapist.

Included within the YEIS is an 11 week (school term) **Youth Transitional Programme** (YTP) that includes an occupational therapist and teacher of education. The programme aim is to promote successful return to school or work and has three components: education vocational support; groups that include stress management, life skills, fitness, and recreational activities; and family involvement in the process.

Youth Forensic Service (YFS)

This inter-related service provides a specialist service that includes consultations with agencies, screening and mental health assessments, written reports and recommendations to all youth courts in Auckland City. It targets young offenders under the age of 17 years who come in contact with the law. This team has four multidisciplinary professionals who may consult with a CCAFS occupational therapist when necessary.

Liaison with Child and Family Unit (CFU) Starship Children's Hospital

CFU is an 8-bed inpatient and a 15-day patient service for children and adolescents up to the age of 17 years. It provides multidisciplinary team intervention that includes a full-time occupational therapist, and has an on site schoolroom for both primary and secondary school pupils. The occupational therapist, clinically responsible to CFU, liaises with CCAFS for professional support. The role is primarily consultative with clinical emphasis on assessment, supervision of groups and specific group work, i.e. process-oriented problem solving and activity groups.

CFU Triple A Team

The CFU includes a team of four professionals with expertise in Autism Spectrum Disorders. The Autism and Asperger Assessment team (Triple A Team) includes an occupational therapist as coordinator and consultant (Christie, 1999). It operates one day a week and deals with children who present with complex, multifaceted autistic spectrum problems, and their families. It is temporarily in abeyance while waiting further funding.

---

address psychosocial and emotional development in children. More recently occupational therapy literature has begun to address this area of need (Cronin 1996, Kramer & Hinojosa 1993, Lewin & Reed 1998, Mosey 1986, Parham & Fazio 1997, Wilcock 1998, Yerxa 1994). These and other sources of literature (Barkley 1998a,b, Bloomquist 1996, Sattler 1989) together with the 'Uniform terminology for occupational therapy' (American Occupational Therapy Association 1994), are used to compile occupational therapy checklists in order to address this area of need in assessment and intervention. Use is made, for example, of classroom and playground observational checklists, social and emotional developmental checklists, group intervention checklists on play and social skills to monitor outcomes.

Intervention may be individual using a variety of theories, models of practice and frames of reference (see Box 13.1) or group oriented (Box 13.5). The clinical emphasis is on using legitimate tools of practice such as the non-human environment, conscious use of self, teaching–learning process, purposeful activities, activity groups, activity analysis and synthesis. Play theory, sensory integration procedures, behavioural, social and emotional learning theories, knowledge of normal child development and family systems are found to be useful approaches. When appropriate, parents, teachers or care-givers are involved in intervention as 'co-therapists', assisting the therapist to meet shared objectives. School or home programmes always support intervention.

.5 List of CCAFS specific group interventions

arenting groups

Challenging Children and Parenting Group (CCAP)

This is a structured four-session group with a parent manual (Christie & Hedayati 1998) that provides learning objectives, homework and information on child development and behaviour (Dinkmeyer & McKay 1989). It is evaluated by the TELER (Le Roux 1998) system.

YEIS Parent Support Group

Provides opportunities for parents to share their experiences of having a child with a mental health illness in a safe environment. There is a psychoeducational component that includes information on a variety of topics such as medication, symptoms, adolescent development and behaviour. The group convenes every 6 weeks.

Pacific Island Parent Support Group (PIPS)

This is a cultural group of mixed Pacific Island peoples. Facilitated by CCAFS Pacific Island cultural adviser, it addresses the issues of parenting and child management in the New Zealand culture and the sharing of mixed cultural experiences.

Maori Women's Support Group

This group is available for Maori mothers of children and youth who have mental health issues. It is informal and attempts to address the cultural and spiritual differences between the Maori and Pakeha perspectives of mental health.

Play groups

The 'Dinosaur Club' is for children aged 5–7 years. It is small (four to six participants), short term (six sessions), and focuses on play (Parham & Fazio 1997) and prosocial skills (Bloomquist 1996). The protocol incorporates a pre-course meeting to assist parents in understanding children's play. The manual (Bailey 1998) provides play information for parents, learning objectives and homework.

Social interaction groups

The social interaction group protocol (Christie 1998) divides children into four developmental levels of social competence (Cartledge & Milburn 1996, Hutchings, Comins & Offiler 1995) from ages 8 to 16 years. Group manuals contain social skills information, activities and homework (Christie 1996). Pre- and post-course meetings focus on psychosocial education, videos and social problem-solving strategies for parents. Videoing and the TELER (Le Roux 1998) system achieve evaluation results. There are two group focuses.

1. Children who have impaired social cognition and perception (i.e. autistic spectrum and pervasive developmental disorders). Small structured (two or three participants) groups that are content specific (Dalrymple 1992, Gray 1994, Quill 1995). Social learning is supported by the parents and schools, and may involve normal peer modelling.

2. Children who have impaired social mastery and intrinsic motivation (i.e. attention deficit/hyperactivity disorder (ADHD), anxiety disorders, post-traumatic stress syndrome) (Barker 1998a,b, Bloomquist 1996, Doble & Magill-Evans 1992) attend groups that are small (six to eight participants) and short term (six sessions). Teachers and parents are involved in completing pre- and post-social skill evaluations (Fernando & Christie 1991a,b) to monitor short- and long-term changes.

Adolescent social skills group

'How to win friends and influence people' is a small structured group for adolescents (14–18 years) who have experienced a first episode of psychosis, bipolar affective disorder or obsessive–compulsive disorder. The objective is to increase social confidence (Kelly 1996); a self-evaluation process is used. The group operates weekly for six sessions.

Stress management group

Developed for young teenage women (13–16 years) who have self-harmed, borderline personality disorder or anxiety problems. The group uses a cognitive-behavioural approach and runs for 12 sessions (Hedayati & Grohman 1998). It aims to develop self-efficacy, extend the repertoire of coping strategies, and provide opportunities for support and shared experiences.

Pizza group

A 'club' model catering for the YEIS adolescent (13–18 years) client group. It runs bimonthly and includes psychoeducational activities, is activity based and provides decision-making opportunities.

Sibling groups

A supportive 'club' model group for brothers and sisters of children with mental health issues. It provides psychoeducation, a developmental and problem-solving perspective, and is focused towards children aged 12 years and above.

Generic role of the therapist in CCAFS

In New Zealand multidisciplinary team-based practice presents a challenge for occupational therapists. They need to be proactive within a team of people who may lack understanding of occupational therapy (Christie 1999b). CCAFS policy is for professionals to work in pairs. The occupational therapist works across disciplines, gaining understanding of different roles and expertise, sharing knowledge, and making decisions about intervention with team support. Approximately 50% of a therapist's time may be devoted to individual clinical and group work, and 50% to generic and service project tasks that include clinical and managerial aspects. This proportion is dependent on the experience of the therapist, for example a new graduate would devote more time to clinical training and less on generic tasks.

Team members are expected to develop expertise in various generic functions. The CCAFS team, supporting mental health facilities and community agencies, provides training in these tasks (Box 13.6).

Box 13.6 Generic tasks of occupational therapists in the CCAFS team

Crisis intervention

Assessment of self-harm attempts and related crises that include administering assessments outside the usual criteria of occupational therapy (American Psychiatric Association 1994, Sattler, 1989).

Service development projects

Includes developing and presenting educational and training packages for community settings, medics, postgraduates, students; research; service provision (i.e. developing assessment and intervention ADHD (CCAFS 1996) and autism protocols, social interaction group protocols); quality assurance subgroup; parent and child information packages.

Computer literacy

Knowledge of database, word processing and publishing are essential skills (Christie & Marsh 1988a,b).

Contribution

To journal clubs, inservices, team building and staff training.

CCAFS service provision processes

Diagnostic interviewing techniques (Sattler 1998) and allocation, review and case management processes (CCAFS 1996).

Specific occupational therapy role

Role development requires therapists to identify their particular skills and knowledge within the team and to understand the unique contribution they can make to successful outcomes for the client (Christie 1999b). The American Occupational Therapy Association's (1994) uniform terminology system defines the paradigm for occupational therapy with performance areas, components and contexts providing the focus for service provision (NZAOT 1992). Occupational performances are strongly influenced by a person's age, stage of development, sociocultural background and environment (Christiansen & Baum 1991, Kramer & Hinojosa 1993), in particular the psychosocial aspects that constitute the performance components of sensory integration (Fisher, Murray & Bundy 1991), cognitive and psychological function, and social interaction (Cronin 1996). This includes the five subdivisions of (1) occupational performance, (2) family interaction (Barker 1992, Corey 1982), (3) school (Dunn 1991), (4) work and play (Parham & Fazio 1997), and (5) leisure, recreation and temporal adaptation (Case-Smith, Allen & Pratt 1996, Creek, 1990), and refers to the social roles of children (Mosey 1986). In addition, family systems approach (Humprey & Case-Smith 1996) and cultural perspective (Fernando 1991) are emphasised.

Box 13.7 describes CCAFS intervention where the therapist worked in association with a multidisciplinary team colleague and as the case manager.

An 'Occupational therapy student learning objectives manual' has been developed to support third year occupational therapy students. It contains site-specific, practical learning experiences (Christie & Doe 1995), opportunities to develop skill in the application of theoretical knowledge, and clinical reasoning through real and paper case examples. More importantly, it provides structured supervision for learning to take place.

Occupational therapists are encouraged to present at conferences (Christie 1997, 1998, Scaletti & Christie 1996), to write for publications

---

Box 13.7 Case example: Ian

Ian is a 6-year-old boy who has elective mutism. He has not spoken for 3 years, but is known to whisper sometimes to his mother. Language-based tests and assessments were inappropriate and had already proved unhelpful at school. Two professionals, an art therapist and an occupational therapist, saw the child and family separately and together, and set objectives with the family, child and school. The therapists shared their individual objectives and outcomes, adapting the programmes where appropriate to meet the child's needs.

The art therapist held individual sessions on site. The occupational therapist undertook the consulting role, performing classroom and home clinical observations, implementing carefully designed programmes for teachers and parents. These programmes consisted of psychoeducation on elective mutism and the developmental implications for Ian (i.e. impaired social and emotional learning). A tape recorder monitored his whispered reading exercises at home. In the classroom visual strategy charts assisted and promoted functional communication (Hodgdon 1995, Quill 1995). By means of play, Ian was encouraged to express emotions, initially non-verbally then verbally, through the use of board and card games in which the whole class was eventually involved.

This integrated focus across settings produced a change for the child and family. Ian started to speak, first at home, and then gradually in class. Social interaction skills were addressed individually at first, then in a small playgroup, and finally, as mastery improved, he attended one of the on-site social skill groups. This final group was supported in the classroom and playground through the use of a 'buddy system'.

---

and to undertake research projects. A longitudinal study of Katie, a child with autism (Christie & Robertson 1991, 1993), is in progress following development from the age of 22 months to 11 years. A further paper is planned to document middle childhood and adolescent years.

Youth Early Intervention Service

Over the past 4 years New Zealand has established services based on an 'early intervention' model, which involves the detection of early psychosis and the provision of specialist, comprehensive treatment aimed to prevent chronic illness (Whitehorn, Lazier & Kopala 1998). The CCAFS-interrelated YEIS is an example of an early psychosis service and includes an occupational therapist in the team of four people. The service provides assertive case management and biopsychosocial interventions for young people aged 15–18 years and their families.

The role of the occupational therapist in Early Psychosis services is not well documented in the literature. The YEIS clinical role focuses on specific occupational therapy assessments and provision of individual and group interventions, primarily in the pre-psychotic and recovery phases of the illness. During the acute phase, the adolescent is usually admitted to the CFU Service.

It is during adolescence that the expectation for independence and self-sufficiency in occupational and social role performance increases. However, the onset of psychosis often disrupts the person's ability to perform competently (Henry & Coster 1996), with many young people dropping out of school and often losing contact with friends and family. Occupational therapy offers individual and group interventions to assist young people to return to previous social, vocational and educational activities. Assessment and treatment is primarily structured using the Canadian Occupational Performance Model (Townsend et al 1997) and the Model of Human Occupation (Kielhofner 1985) and other psychosocial frames of reference (Borg & Bruce 1993).

Box 13.8 describes a YEIS occupational therapy intervention with a young adolescent female following an acute admission to the CFU at Starship Children's Hospital.

Box 13.8 Case example: Karen

Karen, a 16-year-old young woman, was referred to YEIS during an admission to the CFU Starship Children's Hospital with a first presentation of psychosis. The CFU occupational therapist discovered that she would like to leave school and find employment, but was unsure of what direction to take.

Assessment included the Occupational Performance History Interview (Kielhofner & Henry 1988), the Canadian Occupational Performance Measure (Law, Baptiste, Carswell, McColl, Polatajko & Pollock 1994) and an Interest Checklist (CCAFS 1996). These assessments identified a supportive family background, Karen's strengths included a sense of humour, her willingness to learn, and an interest in people.

On consultation between both therapists it was agreed that Karen would participate in the CFU occupational therapy programmes and the YEIS occupational therapist would undertake the long-term vocational plans for Karen. The aim of YEIS is to support adolescents with severe mental health issues for a period of two years. An integral part of this provision was for Karen and her family to learn about the vocational rehabilitation aspect of occupational therapy and the Youth Transitional Programme (YTP) (see Box 13.4). It was explained that the YTP was an 11-week, goal-oriented programme to facilitate reintegration into the community, either school or vocational schemes, and that Karen met the entry criteria for this programme.

The programme assisted Karen to develop a career pathway with steps to show achievement. Her long-term vocational goal was to work in the hospitality industry and as a second option, office administration. The short-term goals were implemented through the programme.

1. To participating in the programme activities of:

   • Focus groups, i.e. stress management skills

   • Life skills group, i.e. psycho-education sessions on the nature and effects of mental health difficulties

   • Fitness for fun activities that include various sports, i.e. swimming

   • Leisure and recreation pursuits, i.e. photography.

2. To investigate courses in hospitality and office administration.

   Karen volunteered to assist with the programme's administration, using her previously learnt typing skills to keep records, design posters, timetables and information leaflets. In addition she willingly participated in the activities where she demonstrated improved self-esteem, confidence and an emerging ability to self-monitor her health needs.

   The next step involved researching career courses and discussing options with her family and therapist. At the completion of the YTP Karen secured a place on a 26-week Skills New Zealand course that would give her the foundation for entry into a hospitality course run by a local technical institute in the year 2001.

Group intervention

Groups are a major part of clinical practice and cater for a range of ages. Two professionals facilitate each group. The occupational therapy role includes consultation, planning and facilitating these groups with another team member (Corey 1982, Sattler 1998). Although model driven, approaches tend to be eclectic, reflecting the knowledge of both professionals, and have skill acquisition, problem resolution, and explorative or psychodynamic psychotherapy components. The group protocols have clear objectives, an evaluation process (Le Roux 1998), with participant manuals supporting many of the groups. The group protocols (Christie 1998) and support manuals (Christie 1996, 1999a, Christie & Hedayati 1998) of the two longest operating groups – CCAP (13 years) and the social skills group (8 years) – were developed by the occupational therapist (Christie 1999b) and are continually upgraded to meet the needs of children and families. These concepts are now used in the planning of new groups.

Service development projects

Four projects involving occupational therapists are currently being implemented. Divided into developmental groupings, they target areas of need as identified by the CCAFS and the Mason Inquiry (1996) (see Box 13.9). One of these projects aims to target the children of our increasing refugee and migrant population. The New Zealand government has established a quota system for refugees, taking 750 each year, many of whom remain in the Auckland area. The psychological complexities arising from the effects of trauma for refugees (Eisenbruch 1991, Bremner 1995) makes them more vulnerable to mental health problems and has become an increasing concern for the CCAFS team.

Box 13.9 Service development projects that involve occupational therapy

Project 1 (0–5 years)

This project targets disruptive behaviour and reactive attachment disorder client groups (Weider 1995). It includes maternal mental health difficulties and the recognised risk factors linked to development and persistence of problem behaviours in preschool aged children. The programme provides home-based assessment, support and modelling of parenting, education on early childhood development, parenting practices, coping strategies and problem-solving skills.

Project 2 (5–12 years)

The Schools Liaison Project (SLIP) is a school-based programme using a consultation model of practice that provides assessment, consultation, training and psycho-education for school staff in the difference between mental health issues and the three identified mental health disorders. The targeted areas include the three predominant diagnostic groups for children between the ages of 5 and 12 years; disruptive disorders, pervasive developmental disorders, anxiety and mood disorders. School-based clinics aim to support existing clients and identify those children in need of assessment and intervention. This pilot project involving four schools was conducted in 1999 with the programme extending to other schools in the year 2000. The project leader is a senior occupational therapist.

Project 3 (13 + years)

The Liaison and Education Adolescent Project (LEAP), using a consultation model of practice, extends current service provision to schools, community agencies and general practitioners. The aims are to improve access and resources. It provides liaison and collaboration to agencies, psycho-education workshops, and increased knowledge base and research of CCAFS on the adolescent mental health issues targeted by LEAP. These identified areas include depression, anxiety, conduct disorder, obsessive–compulsive disorder, bipolar affective disorder, psychosis, borderline personality and post-traumatic stress disorder.

Project 4 (children of refugees)

This project aims to provide a specialist service for children and adolescents of refugee and migrant families who are experiencing mental health problems arising from trauma and disruption.

The projects have set objectives and outcomes that will determine future service provision planning. It is envisaged that these projects could evolve into interrelated services (e.g. the SLIP project) and improve the efficiency of the community team for children, their families and supporting agencies.

CHILD AND FAMILY SERVICES IN THE COMMUNITY: A NON-GOVERNMENT AGENCY

Rowena Scaletti

In response to the changing demands of the health service in New Zealand, and the increasingly generic nature of health professionals, occupational therapists are moving away from traditional hospital-based service delivery into the community. There is a large network of multidisciplinary and cross-cultural agencies, large and small, working in the community, with a variety of team compositions. These agencies are accountable firstly to their own Boards and Social Services, and secondly to central government if they wish to retain some government funding through the New Zealand Community Funding Agency (CFA).

One example of community-based child, adolescent, and family mental health service is the non-government organisation (NGO), where, although professional qualifications are acknowledged and valued, employment is predominantly generic, or skill based.

The following discussion describes one such role undertaken by an occupational therapist as a counsellor/therapist in such an organisation, or agency, in a low socioeconomic and culturally diverse area of Auckland, New Zealand's largest city. The agency, Baptist Action Family Services, is a child and family support service focused on servicing children and families experiencing abuse, neglect or disruption. The agency endeavours to provide a quality service that ensures the safety of children, is culturally appropriate wherever possible, and strengthens families/whanau.

Location

The wider service, or agency, includes six teams addressing particular community needs (see Box 13.10) and is situated in a suburban street. It is easily accessed by train and bus services, with off-street parking. Apart from administration and the counselling team (which works from an elderly wisteria and jasmine-covered villa), the other teams work mainly in the community and clients' homes, with office space provided on site.

Referrals

Referrals for counselling come from a variety of sources, the data-gathering system in place within the agency using a common format for all teams (Fig. 13.1). Most requests come directly from a con-

INWARD FORM

THERAPIST:

CLIENT: REFERRAL DATE:

REFERRAL SOURCE: (circle letter)

A	CYPS	Papakura
B	CYPS	Otara
C	CYPS	Mangere
D	CYPS	Other:
E	Police/Justice system	
F	Health services/Plunket/Hospitals/GPs	
G	Education services	
H	Other organisation:	
I	Friend/Family	
J	Self	
K	Marae/Cultural group	

PRIMARY FAMILY PROBLEM: (circle letter)

A   Sexual abuse
B   Physical abuse
C   Care-giver/s unwilling/unable to care for CYP
D   Conflict between CYP and care-giver
E   Inability to deal with CYP behavioural problems
F   Insufficient resources to meet needs of CYP
G   Other:

SERVICES PROVIDED: A   Counselling/Family therapy

ETHNICITY: (circle letter)

M   Maori
P   Pakena
S   Samoan
T   Tongan
R   Rarotongan/Cook Island
N   Nulean
F   Fijian
A   Asian
X   Other:

IWI AFFILIATION:

GEOGRAPHICAL AREA: (circle number)

1 Manurewa	2 Papakura	3 Manukau	4 Otara
5 Mangere	6 Pukekohe	7 Howlek	8 Papatoetoe
Other			

GENDER: (circle letter)

M – Male   F – Female   X – Family

Figure 13.1   Agency inward form/referral source. CYPS, Children and Young Persons Service; CYP, child or young person; GP, general practitioner.

Box 13.10 Non-government agency: breakdown by teams

1. Administration: a supportive service for all teams, and liaison with other agencies.

2. Counselling service: a solution-oriented approach to change for families experiencing conflict and disruptions in their lives

3. Homebuilders team: a home-based family support service which enables families to function well and remain together.

4. Parent support team: a home-based crisis intervention service for families with young children whose parents/care-givers are temporarily unable to cope because of sickness, accident, crisis or trauma.

5. Social work team: to provide alternative care for families under stress; to provide an advocacy service for families; to support families and Family Homes; to liaise with statutory agencies, such as the police, and the Department of Child, Youth and Family Service.

6. Supervised access team: a multicultural service for separated families providing an independent, safe and neutral setting for parents and children to interact and play.

Box 13.11 Types of problem referred

- abuse
- anger
- behavioural problems
- domestic violence
- family conflict
- grief and loss
- separated families
- stepfamily issues

---

cerned family member, frequently the mother. Most commonly a family/whanau relationship approach (New Zealand CFA 1998) is the first response (50%) to all referred issues, the main exception being young persons, those aged 16 years and under, who frequently receive individual counselling. It is the policy of the counselling team to meet with the whole family at the initial assessment, unless there are issues of safety. 'Family' is defined by those requesting counselling and may include people who are there to provide a cultural perspective, is close and supportive, but not necessarily related in the usual sense.

Types of problem referred

The clinical approach is generic, not medical; therefore, families are encouraged to understand that a problem affects everyone, not one particular family member. The approach is descriptive not diagnostic. When medical advice is needed, families are advised to visit their family doctor, who will be encouraged to liaise with the counsellor/therapist. The types of problems typically seen at the counselling centre (see Box 13.11) are

addressed within a systemic family approach, with concurrent individual or group therapy as needed.

Main treatment approaches

A generic rather than medical approach has determined the need to build a partnership with families to resolve problems. The ethical issues of power and control in therapeutic relationships preclude the image of one person 'treating' another. An agreement with the family is reached concerning their needs, and their acceptance (or not) of what the counsellor/therapist is able to offer in terms of the change process. The engagement of the family in a partnership for change at the first meeting means an acceptance and understanding that what affects one affects all. The means for change are based within a family therapy approach, with the use of associated therapies to address particular individual needs (see Box 13.1).

Counselling team

The counselling team has four members at present, working a total of 120 hours weekly. The composition of the team changes with staff turnover, but may consist of staff with backgrounds in education, nursing, occupational therapy, psychology or social work. All have skills and qualifications in individual and family therapy. The various skills brought to the team provide a broad and strong therapy base from which the team works.

The counselling team also takes responsibility for supervising students on clinical placement, together with lecturing to students at institutes of technology. Mounting seminars and hui (cultural meeting), developing new initiatives, as well as liaising with agency teams, community groups and schools, form an important part of the team's role.

To illustrate how the generic approach to change is melded with occupational therapy theory, three case studies are described and analysed. Names and some clinical details have been altered to ensure confidentiality and anonymity.

The generic role of the occupational therapist

Many children experience emotional distress or trauma, which may affect not only them but also the entire family structure. This may occur, for example, through parental separation or death, domestic violence, abuse, or personal disfigurement from burns, amputation or injury. Children's occupational behaviour, or how they perform their day-to-day tasks and activities, is frequently the first indicator of emotional distress. Behavioural changes, including aggression, withdrawal, distress and refusal to take part in previously enjoyed activities, are common (Gil 1991). How children cope with and adapt to emotional distress influences the development of their concept of self (Brewer 1998, Gilhotra 1995), as well as the process of learning and manner of social interaction (Scaletti 1999). It is upon such outcomes that lives and life chances are built. The continuity of role development in childhood is dependent on children's ability to interact with family and peers in a variety of social, learning and developmental situations (Olson 1993).

CASE STUDY 1:   PLAY AND THE NARRATIVE APPROACH TO FAMILY THERAPY

Play, innate to children (Vandenberg & Kielhofner 1982), and frequently considered their most important occupation (Larsen 1995), provides a strong therapeutic medium for emotionally disturbed children (Bentovim 1977, Smith 1977). Through the suspension of reality, play creates opportunities for children to project their anxiety and transform fantasies into communication (Gavshon 1989), and encourages the return to, or development of, the occupational behaviours of childhood incorporated within family and social life (Olson 1993).

Behaviour is frequently determined by meanings attributed to experience (White 1989–1991) and, as E. Bruner (1986) and J. Bruner (1987) have described, there are many aspects of lived experience that are neglected when a problem story is told. Dominant problem-saturated stories, which are by definition selective of experience (Zimmerman & Dickerson 1994), are created through people's perceptions and subjective realities. The narrative metaphor, by emphasising order and sequence (Gergen & Gergen 1984), becomes the means for reshaping or re-authoring people's stories over time. The use of language and questioning encourages people to describe their own experiences, not others' descriptions of their experiences (White 1989–1990). The narrative approach, through the sharing of power and the use of child-oriented language, enables people to become their own catalyst for change (Epston 1993).

The practice of externalising problem stories (White & Epston 1990) addresses the common Western practice of objectifying people. When children are angry, they are frequently labelled as being conduct disordered, as attention deficit, or oppositional. Some children may be seen as the cause of a sibling's unacceptable behaviour, or family's dysfunction. Externalisation changes the relationship between the person and the problem, freeing the person from those cultural practices that locate the problem within the person or relationship. The problem is relocated within the social and sociopolitical context (Madigan 1992), the problem and its sphere of influence being identified as the problem, not the person or their relationships. That is, the problem is the problem.

A child's innate ability to create fantasy play to rewrite the problem story through narrative metaphor (Burke & Schaaf 1997, Fazio 1991) uses alternative untold stories to break the power of the problem. It becomes unnecessary to find the cause of the problem, or who is to blame, thus removing feelings of powerlessness and blame, freeing the family to unite in vanquishing the foe.

Example: Tom and his battle with LOSING TEMPER

Tom, a 6-year-old boy, is the only child of a sole parent. After the death of his grandfather, he continued to live with his mother and semi-invalid grandmother. Tom's schoolteacher referred him for counselling for increasingly aggressive behaviour. Tom's feelings of loss and grief following the death of his grandfather, and the impact of these changes on the family structure, were thought to have precipitated the behavioural changes.

The process

Relative influence questioning.   The first meeting and interview with Tom and his mother focused on questions that engaged them in the process of separating their lives and relationships from the problem (White 1988). From a broad description of the problem that was affecting their family life (i.e. Tom's angry and aggressive behaviour) came strategies that could be used to take action against the problem. The purpose was to empower the family in their control over the problem, not to eliminate the problem entirely.

Mapping the influence of persons on the problem.   Once the family has mapped the influence of the problem over their lives, they are asked to recall times they have influenced the life of the problem. Questions and creative play are used to discover how they have managed to resist giving in to the power of the problem, and what strengths they were able to use.

Occupational behaviour.   Tom and his mother recalled times when Tom had been able to resist the power of the problem. They were able to recall many instances, some of which had been noticed by Tom's grandmother and his teacher.

Questions around resistance encourage the family to create an externalised description of the problem, and come to an alternative view of events. Time is collapsed, and the life of the problem placed in a temporal context. Trends of influence, often imperceptible until gathered during questioning, are used to show distinctions or differences between the strength and power of the problem at opposing times. These inconsistencies underlie change.

Defining the problem to be externalised.   The family is encouraged to talk about the problem in terms of separateness and difference from the person or relationship to which it is seen to belong. The problem is personified, that is, named and drawn or described by the child. The process opens up new ways for an attack on the problem.

Tom decided to call the problem LOSING TEMPER, and drew a large scary monster with horns, which came into his home and made trouble for everyone. Tom's mother said they always knew when LOSING TEMPER was hanging around because of the power it had over Tom.

Unique outcomes.   Those sparkling moments when the family has been able to resist an invitation to join with the problem, and the meanings attached to them, become the impetus for change. Family members are invited to recall moments of resistance, current or historical, that have minimised the power of the problem.

Occupational role.   Tom and his mother were asked to identify how LOSING TEMPER influenced Tom's behaviour and feelings, as well as his occupational roles of student, son, grandson and peer. They described how LOSING TEMPER was taking over Tom's social interactions and attitudes (White & Epston 1990), and came to realise the ways in which they had unknowingly kept LOSING TEMPER alive (White 1986). Tom, however, did remember the time when he was able to punch LOSING TEMPER on the nose, kick it in the shins, and shut it outside the bedroom while he tidied up. Suddenly, Tom's mother noticed how Tom was talking about the power LOSING TEMPER had over him at home and school without getting defensive and angry. Everyone wondered how Tom managed this.

Unique outcomes and creative play.   The use of creative play, ritual and imagination assists the process of externalisation and aids identification of unique outcomes. It is essential for the therapist to use what is significant for the family.

Sense of self.   Tom's relationship with LOSING TEMPER was weakening but Tom still worried about being beaten. A meeting of Tom's team

(Tom, mum, therapist) worked out how to trap LOSING TEMPER in a box. Tom raced around and caught LOSING TEMPER and stuffed it in a box. LOSING TEMPER fought and fought, but the team got the box shut and tied up. The therapist said she would put it on her shelf and watch over it.

Tom's sense of who he is, his self-esteem and self-concept (Mayberry 1990) becomes less and less determined by how he behaves. He is enabled to make choices of his own, to rewrite his own story.

Revision of a person's relationship with the problem: predicting relapses

Interdependence between the problem and its effects is essential for the problem's survival. As families work toward creating a different story, which lessens this interdependence, relapses will inevitably occur. These expected events, often reframed as hiccups or counterplots, provide ways of knowing what types of resistance, or unique outcomes, sever the relationship with the problem.

Responsibilities

Externalisation of the problem gives people greater choice and power over problem domination of their lives. Rather than evading responsibility for the problem, it provides a sense of freedom with the knowledge that they are able to act independently of the problem.

Spreading the good news: re-creation of the self

Every good story needs an audience. The more it is enacted, told or read, the more real it becomes. Power is shared throughout the process of change, as the emerging story is re-enacted through creative and fantasy play. It may be documented in letters from the therapist to the child. The re-authoring of a person's story, with its beginning, middle and end, belongs to the person.

During Tom's visits to the therapist, everyone would talk about the time when Tom would be ready to finish off LOSING TEMPER for good.

The day came when Tom and his mother decided that LOSING TEMPER hardly ever came around to their house any more. The therapist took the secure box with LOSING TEMPER outside, where Tom jumped and jumped on it, shouting and yelling at LOSING TEMPER that he was not to come any more. LOSING TEMPER struggled, but eventually Tom was the winner.

Liberation

The therapist awarded Tom a certificate for beating LOSING TEMPER, and Tom thought he could tell other children how he had managed this. LOSING TEMPER did try to come around to Tom's house from time to time, but Tom and his mother were always ready for him.

Graduation from the tyranny of the problem is often ritually celebrated: a final letter, shared food and drink, an award. Many cultures celebrate important life changes. A new life deserves no less.

Through a family-centred narrative approach, the child is part of a social group, not a diagnosis. Stories and metaphors provide a pathway for therapists and families to walk together in the resolution of childhood behavioural problems (Burke & Schaaf 1997, Fazio 1991, Henley 1994, Park 1982) and the development of occupational behaviour. Through intrinsic motivation embedded in play (Morrison, Metzger & Pratt 1996), playfulness (Bundy 1997) and the use of fantasy and creative play, children are enabled to develop a sense of social mastery (Cronin 1996) which forms the basis for those innate behavioural and social adjustments that are essential for day-to-day living in the social arena.

CASE STUDY 2: PSYCHOSOCIAL DEVELOPMENT, CHILDREN'S GROUPS AND DOMESTIC VIOLENCE

The acknowledgement of domestic violence as a criminal act in New Zealand (New Zealand Government 1996) and the subsequent availability of funds for counselling for both protected persons and respondents (the offenders) has enabled many families to seek help through counselling. In the context of the New Zealand Domestic Violence Act 1995, domestic violence includes physical abuse, sexual abuse and damage to property. It also stipulates 'psychological abuse, including but not limited to intimidation, harassment, damage to property, threats of physical abuse, sexual abuse, or causing or allowing the child to see or hear the physical, sexual, or psychological abuse of a person with whom the child has a domestic relationship' (p. 8). The Act states 'a single act may amount to abuse, or a number of acts that form a pattern of behaviour . . . even though some or all of the acts, when viewed in isolation, may appear to be minor or trivial' (pp. 8–9).

Occupational therapy views the individual as performing activities and roles within a social, cultural and physical environment, with occupational performance reflecting the individual's dynamic experience (Baum 1995). The behaviour of children affected by domestic violence is generally reflective of the fear, insecurity and hypervigilance (Briere 1996, Ericksen & Henderson 1992, Maxwell 1994, Maxwell & Carroll-Lind 1996, Vissing et al 1991) associated with violence in the home. The impact on child development may show as signs of anxious attachment, withdrawal from social relationships, aggressive and/or controlling behaviour (Jaffe, Wolfe & Wilson 1990, National Clearinghouse on Family Violence 1995, Pocock & Cram 1996, Wright 1994). The need to reconcile feelings of attachment and love, with fear and withdrawal from a violent and previously loved and trusted person, can cause confusion, anger and a generalised mistrust. For children, like adults, the opportunity to share their feelings with those who have similar experiences provides a 'safe place' to learn different ways of coping with anger, loss and emotional pain (Olson 1993, Pfeifer 1992). The provision of a 'safe place', or group, where children can be encouraged through structured play, creativity and fun to share their experiences with others who have had similar experiences (Frey-Angel 1989, Kemp & Milne 1997, Smith & Sparks 1995, Scaletti & Tolley

1998), becomes an essential part of their recovery process. Children are secondary victims no more.

The counselling team offers three group approaches to working with those affected by domestic violence:

1. Family groups for children and the custodial parent
2. Sibling groups for children in a foster-care situation
3. Age-related groups, or clubs, for children, with the custodial parent attending three concurrent parent meetings.

The purpose of each group is to help children and their families cope with the effects of family violence. The extensive manual developed by Scaletti & Tolley (1998), and approved by the New Zealand Department of Courts, provides an effective content, process and reference source. It sets out the theoretical rationale, assessments and procedures for all types of group.

The following discussion presents an example of the content (Table 13.1), together with process and outcome goals (Fig. 13.2), of the children's age-related group: 5–7, 8–10 and 11–12 years.

Example: Kids Feeling Safe Groups

Children's clubs, or Kids Feeling Safe groups, were started in 1998 in response to the growing awareness of families showing the effects of domestic violence on their lives and relationships. Children referred for inclusion in a club are assessed by one of the group facilitators. This includes an initial assessment of the history of domestic violence from the parent/care-giver, and the degree of post-traumatic stress experienced by the child (Briere 1996). The ability of the child to talk about their memories of the violence, how they feel about it, and contain their behaviour to some extent, is essential. It is at this screening interview that children are either accepted into a club or referred for individual therapy. An exit assessment is made within 1 month of club finishing. At this time, decisions

Table 13.1   Example of group content for session 5: anger and conflict resolution

Time	Action	Person	Equipment
10 min	Welcome Karakia and afternoon tea Review club rules and last week's content		Welcome chart Drinks and food Club rules chart
10 min	Feelings check-in Each child uses their name tag to name today's feeling – 'I feel . . . because . . .'		Feelings chart Name tags
15 min	Anger: children draw pictures about anger, naming what is happening, when it happens, and how it feels 'A time when I felt angry'		Felt pens Paper
15 min	Social skills and social relationships Interactive team-building game		Playground Follow the leader
15 min	Brainstorm: what we might do if we were angry Puppets: children and facilitators role-play with puppets, showing ways of managing anger in abusive and non-abusive ways		Paper and pens Puppets
10 min	Closure: one of the children reads out the letter to parent/care-giver Goodbye circle – multilingual goodbyes		Letter Goodbye chart

From Scaletti & Tolley (1998).

are made concerning further therapy, individual or family, intermittent follow-up or closure.

The children's clubs are run over a period of 8 weeks, each session taking $1\frac{1}{4}$ hours. The content and process of the club are designed to create confidence and self-esteem, together with the knowledge that all forms of abuse are wrong and not the child's fault. A psychoeducational approach is taken, combined with creative art activities and play, frequently using puppets. The process is essentially one of empowerment through knowledge and understanding.

The topics addressed throughout the 8-week course (see Box 13.12) are those identified in the New Zealand Domestic Violence Act 1995 as essential to the recovery process. The clubs are multicultural and emphasis is placed on the use of different languages in the greeting and farewell components of the programme. The programme is interactive, the goal being to create a cohesive club culture. The philosophy of the club is that the output of a group is greater than the sum of its parts.

CASE STUDY 3:   PSYCHOSOCIAL DEVELOPMENT, GRIEF AND ATTACHMENT LOSS

With the increasing frequency of loss through family separation, death or violence, many children are referred with anxiety and fear resulting from feelings of rejection or abandonment (Crittenden 1992). The ability of a child to adapt to major assaults on the process of the life cycle

Box 13.12 Weekly topics for aged-based children's groups

Week 1   Getting to know each other and our families
Week 2   Feelings and our support systems
Week 3   Self-esteem and assertiveness
Week 4   Loss and change
Week 5   Anger and conflict resolution
Week 6   Abuse: realistic perspectives
Week 7   Abuse-free ways of relating
Week 8   What we have learned; party and graduation

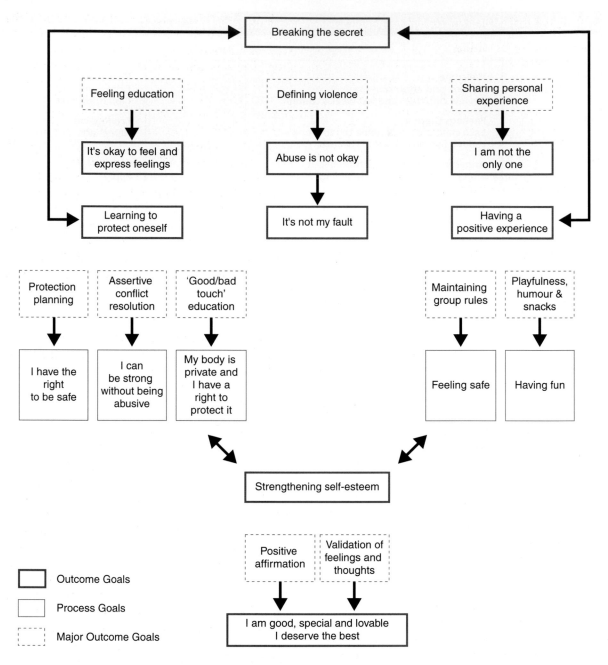

Figure 13.2 Process and outcome goals for Kids Feeling Safe groups. Acknowledgement to: Peled & Davis (1995) Group work with children of battered women.

implies a secure attachment to the remaining parent and their environment (Crittenden 1994). When that parent is themselves grieving their own loss, or later remarries and starts a new family, they sometimes become less available for their child (Byng-Hall 1995).

Example: Sarah

Sarah is a 10-year-old girl whose father died a violent death when she was 2 years old. Her mother then brought her home to New Zealand for the support their extended family could provide. The mother remarried when Sarah was 4 years old, and a further two children were born to the new relationship. Over time Sarah became increasingly moody, clingy with her mother, and behaviourally defiant. This was so out of character that her family referred her for counselling.

The whole family attended the initial interview. They presented as a warm, concerned family. It was observed, however, that Sarah did not join in with the family discussion as readily as other family members. Everyone was encouraged to contribute to the drawing of a family genogram, which included those who had died or were separated from the family. A diagram showing attachment, family ties and alliances was started by the therapist, each member of the family placing themselves in relationship to the others. Sarah drew herself out to the side of the diagram. It was at that time that the mother became aware of her daughter's feelings of abandonment and loss of belonging.

Sarah was seen alone for several sessions. Non-directive play (Cattanach 1994, Furth 1988, McMahon 1992, West 1992) was used as a projective measure to gain Sarah's trust, as well as to allow her to talk and play out her feelings and fears safely. She was able to demonstrate through play her feelings of gradual rejection by her mother as her mother attended to her growing family responsibilities.

The role of Sarah's dead father, and her attachment to him, had become increasingly prominent in her life, as she perceived her mother retreating from her. Sarah thought of him watching over her. She daydreamed how he might come back to the family and everything would be secure again (Black 1998). She wrote letters to him. Together with her drawings, these were left outside for him overnight (Silverman, Nickman & Worden 1992). For Sarah, a fantasy world provided a greater sense of attachment and emotional security than the family she lived with.

Sarah's narrative story became the basis of the change that placed her back within her family. Compiling a photograph album to record her story, she was able to trace her family from before her birth to the present. She wrote letters and poems to her father, and to her mother. These were placed in the album alongside photographs her mother supplied. Through drawings with captions Sarah placed her feelings of loss outside herself, creating a more realistic way of coping.

Special times were set aside for Sarah and mother (Kirkland 1994), halting the gradual emotional and physical divergence between them. When a new baby was born, Sarah became her mother's 'Girl Friday'. The status this provided continued the reclamation of Sarah by her family.

Over time, it became apparent that Sarah's mother had been unable to work through her own feelings of loss, thus contributing to her inability to support Sarah through the violent death of her father. Sarah and her mother found it difficult to speak about their lost father and husband with depth of feeling, thus avoiding acknowledging the true extent of the loss and grief (Neimeyer 1998). Sarah and her mother spent much time talking and crying together. The open realisation of their shared grief and loss became one more strength in their relationship.

The essential need of children to 'belong' in order to progress through normal stages of psychosocial development toward satisfying occupational roles in adulthood is well documented (Donley 1993, Mosey 1981, Olson 1993, Scaletti 1995). Children's affinity for metaphor, creative play and suspension of reality makes play an essential medium for occupational therapy. It is the familiar process of play, often in its projective form, that provides the emotional safety for children to resolve painful experiences. This, in turn, opens up ways for the strengthening of attachments within their family and social worlds.

CONCLUSION

The limited number of occupational therapists working in child and adolescent mental health remains a concern. The use of approved and accredited training manuals, postgraduate internships, together with specific related learning modules, is being considered at present.

The changing political and health systems predict that occupational therapy will continue to adapt in the 21st century. Occupational therapists will also continue to upskill, using external supervision and postgraduate learning to extend their clinical and professional skills. The profession is, however, becoming more consultative and generic. If it is to remain viable, holding to its essential occupational focus, it is essential that a strong mentoring movement, together with the existing NZAOT Cornerstone programme for clinical standards, be pursued. It is also essential that occupational therapists continue to be both professionally and financially accountable.

As Christie (1999b, p. 64) stated: 'As we move toward the millennium it would be encouraging to . . . [look to a system] of mentoring that can inspire, challenge and nurture our professional and clinical pathways to keep our occupational therapy culture alive'.

ADDENDUM

Since this chapter was written, changes continue to influence the development of occupational therapy in child mental health. This is expected to continue. Little specific occupational therapy training is available, therapists tending to undertake complementary professional courses. The University of Auckland Health Science Faculty offers a one-year certificated course or a two-year diploma course in Child and Adolescent Mental Health to clinicians.

CCAFS currently employs 56 people from diverse backgrounds and cultures. Consequently the occupational therapy role has expanded to include a greater number of intervention programmes. In conjunction with psychologists occupational therapists are developing programmes for anxious children as well as those with early mood disorders and the refugee population. A recent development is activity-based programmes for individuals and group work primarily with preschool and middle childhood children. It focuses on the development of social and emotional competence. In addition the consult liaison focus of the SLIP and LEAP projects with schools has encouraged collaborative goal setting between health and education and a greater understanding of child and adolescent mental health disorders.

In the community, increasing demand for counselling services together with diminishing financial support has necessitated a wider programme focus. The core services of trauma counselling for children and families, family therapy, couple counselling, behaviour problems, sibling programmes, domestic violence programmes, and therapy groups for women remain in place. In addition counsellors are developing further group programmes for children. These include integrated therapeutic care for at-risk adolescent boys, children in care, psychoeducation groups for children with psychiatrically disturbed parents, and psychosocial groups for children with sequelae of head injuries, as well as State-funded groups for child and adult survivors of sexual abuse. Consultancy services are to be offered to the community, and existing programmes, such as children's age-based domestic violence programmes, taken into schools.

ACKNOWLEDGEMENTS

The authors gratefully acknowledge contributions from Stephanie Doe NZROT BHSc (occupational therapy) who works at the Early Intervention Centre, West Auckland, and Mathys Lucussen NZROT BHSc (occupational therapy) who works at CCAFS.

REFERENCES

American Occupational Therapy Association 1994 Uniform terminology for occupational therapy, 3rd edn. American Journal of Occupational Therapy 48:1047–1054

American Psychiatric Association 1994 Diagnostic and statistical manual of mental disorders (DSM-IV), 4th edn. American Psychiatric Association, Washington, DC

Attwood A 1997 Asperger's syndrome. Jessica Kingsley, London

Bailey K 1998 Dinosaur club play group manual. Community Child, Adolescent and Family Service, Auckland

Barker P 1992 Basic family therapy, 3rd edn. Blackwell Scientific, London

Barkley R A 1998a Attention deficit hyperactive disorder: a handbook for diagnosis and treatment, 2nd edn. Guilford Press, New York

Barkley R 1998b Attention deficit hyperactive disorder: a clinical workbook. Guilford Press, New York

Baum C 1995 Position paper. Occupational performance: occupational therapy's definition of function. American Journal of Occupational Therapy 49(10): 9–10

Bentovim A 1977 The role of play in psychotherapeutic work with children and their families. In: Tizard B, Harvey D (eds) Biology of play. Heinemann Medical, London, p 185

Black D 1998 Bereavement in childhood. British Medical Journal 316:931–933

Bloomquist M L 1996 Skill training for children with behavior disorders. Guilford Press, New York

Borg B, Bruce M 1993 Psychosocial occupational therapy frames of reference for intervention, 2nd edn. Slack, Thorofare, New Jersey

Bremner J D 1995 Neurobiological implications of posttraumatic stress disorder. National Centre for PTSD, Yale University School of Medicine, New Haven, Connecticut

Brewer P 1998 Efficacy and the self. British Journal of Occupational Therapy 61(5):198–202

Briere J 1996 Trauma symptom checklist for children: professional manual. PAR Psychological Assessments Resources, Boston

Bruner E 1986 Ethnography as narrative. In: Turner V W, Turner E M (eds) The anthropology of experience. University of Illinois Press, Chicago, p 139

Bruner J 1987 Life as narrative. Social Research 54:11–32

Bundy A C 1997 Play and playfulness: what to look for. In: Parham D, Fazio L S (eds) Play in occupational therapy for children. Mosby, St Louis, pp 52–66

Burke J P, Schaaf R C 1997 Family narratives and play assessment. In: Parham D, Fazio L S (eds) Play in occupational therapy for children. Mosby, St Louis, pp 67–84

Byng-Hall J 1995 Creating a secure family base: some implications of attachment theory for family therapy. Family Process 34:45–58

Cartledge G, Milburn J F 1996 Teaching social skills to children and youth: innovative approaches, 2nd edn. Pergamon, London

Case-Smith J, Allen A S, Pratt N P 1996 Occupational therapy for children, 3rd edn. Mosby, Baltimore

Cattanach A 1994 Play therapy. Where the sky meets the underworld. Jessica Kingsley, London

Christiansen C, Baum C (eds) 1991 Occupational therapy: overcoming human performance deficits. Slack, Thorofare, New Jersey

Christie A 1996 Social interaction manual for children. Starship Children's Hospital, Auckland

Christie A 1997 Katie: a child with autism. Unpublished conference paper presented at Making a Difference: Autism Conference Nov 1997 Wellington, NZ

Christie A 1998 A social interaction group protocol. Unpublished conference paper presented at Today's Tomorrow: The Mental Health of Our Tamariki and Rangatahi. The New Zealand Child and Youth Mental Health Conference. Nov 1998 Christchurch, NZ

Christie A 1999a Getting on: a social interaction group manual for children. Auckland-Author

Christie A 1999b New Zealand Association of Occupational Therapists Frances Rutherford lecture. A meaningful occupation: the just right challenge. Australian Occupational Therapy Journal 46:52–68

Christie A, Doe S 1995 Occupational therapy student learning objectives manual. Community Child, Adolescent and Family Service, Auckland

Christie A, Hedayati L 1998 CCAP: challenging children and parenting, 4th edn. Community Child, Adolescent and Family Service, Auckland

Christie A, Marsh S 1988a Computers with the severely disabled: a Sutherland Unit experience. New Zealand Journal of Occupational Therapy 39(1):5–7

Christie A, Marsh S 1988b Computers: a therapeutic tool. New Zealand Journal of Occupational Therapy 40(2): 10–11

Christie A, Robertson S 1991 The use of the Childhood Autism Rating Scale in an occupational therapy programme. New Zealand Journal of Occupational Therapy 42(2):13–16

Christie A, Robertson S 1993 Katie, a child with autism: an occupational therapy case study. New Zealand Journal of Occupational Therapy 44(2):3–10

Collins Concise English Dictionary 1990 2nd edn. William Collins, Glasgow

Community Child, Adolescent and Family Service 1996 Quality assurance protocols for assessment, intervention and review processes. CCAFS, Auckland

Corey G 1982 Theory and practice of counselling and psychotherapy. Brooks Hole, Pacific Grove, California

Creek J 1990 Occupational therapy and mental health: principles, skills and practice. Churchill Livingstone, Edinburgh

Crittenden P M 1992 Children's strategies for coping with adverse home environments: an interpretation using attachment theory. Child Abuse and Neglect 16: 329–343

Crittenden P M 1994 Intimate relationships across the lifespan: implications for personality development. New Zealand Psychological Society Seminar: Ongoing education programme Auckland, New Zealand

Cronin A 1996 Psychosocial and emotional domain of behaviour. In: Case-Smith J, Allen A S, Pratt P N (eds) Occupational therapy for children, 3rd edn. Mosby, St Louis, p 387

Dalrymple N 1992 Some social communication skill objectives and teaching strategies for people with autism. Indiana University, Bloomington, Indiana

Dinkmeyer D, McKay G D 1989 The parents guide: systematic training for effective parenting. American Guidance Service, Circle Pines, Minnesota

Doble S E, Magill-Evans J 1992 A model of social interaction to guide occupational therapy practice. Canadian Journal of Occupational Therapy 59(3): 141–150

Domestic Violence Act 1995 New Zealand Government, Wellington

Donley M G 1993 Attachment and the emotional unit. Family Process 32:3–20

Dunn W 1991 Pediatric occupational therapy: facilitating effective service provision. Slack, Thorofare, New Jersey

Durie M H 1984 'Te Taha Hinengaro': an integrated approach to mental health. Community Mental Health in New Zealand 1(1):4–11

Vandenberg B, Kielhofner G 1982 Play in evolution, culture, and individual adaptation: implications for play. American Journal of Occupational Therapy 36(1):20–28

Vissing Y M, Strauss M A, Gelles R J, Harrop J W 1991 Verbal aggression by parents and psychosocial problems of children. Child Abuse and Neglect 15:223–238

Walker R 1996 People in the Northern Region: a demographic profile from the 1996 census. Health Funding Authority, Auckland

Weider S (ed) 1995 Zero to three: diagnostic classification of mental health and developmental disorders of infancy and early childhood. National Center for Clinical Infant Programs, Arlington, Texas

Werry J S, Scaletti R, Mills F 1990 Sensory integration and teacher-judged learning problems: a controlled intervention trial. Journal of Paediatric Child Health 26:31–35

West J 1992 Child-centred play therapy. Edward Arnold, London

White M 1986 Family escape from trouble. Case Studies 1(1): 29–33

White M 1988 The process of questioning: a therapy of literary merit. Dulwich Centre Newsletter Winter: 8–14

White M 1989–1990 Family therapy training and supervision in a world of experience and narrative. Dulwich Centre Newsletter Summer: 27–38

White M 1989–1991 Deconstruction and therapy. In: Experience, contradiction, narrative and

imagination – selected papers of David Epston & Michael White. Dulwich Centre Publications, Adelaide, p 109

White M, Epston D 1990 Narrative means to therapeutic ends. W W Norton, New York

Whitehead G 1995 Other worlds and other lives: a study of occupational therapy student perceptions of cultural difference. Occupational Therapy International 2:291–313

Whitehorn, D, Lazier L, Kopala L 1998 Psychosocial rehabilitation early after the onset of psychosis. Psychiatric Services 49(9):1135–1146

Wilcock A A 1998 An occupational perspective of health. Slack, Thorofare, New Jersey

Williamson G G, Szczepanski M, Zeitlin S 1993 Coping frame of reference. In: Kramer P, Hinojosa J (eds) Frames of reference for pediatric occupational therapy. Williams & Wilkins, Baltimore, p 395–436

Wright S A 1994 Physical and emotional abuse and neglect of pre-school children: a literature review. Australian Occupational Therapy Journal 41:55–63

Yerxa E J 1994 Dreams, dilemmas, and decisions for occupational therapy practice in the new millennium: an American perspective. American Journal of Occupational Therapy 48:586–589

Zimmerman J L, Dickerson V C 1994 Using a narrative metaphor: implications for theory and clinical practice. Family Process 33:233–245

This section includes two subjects that underpin work in CAMHS. Supervision of practice is essential to all therapists, but, as shown by Sue Evans in Chapter 14, it is acknowledged as necessary to effective clinical practice in CAMHS. Becky Durant tackles the complex subject of the law as it affects children in Chapter 15.

14 Keeping safe: supervision and support

Sue Evans

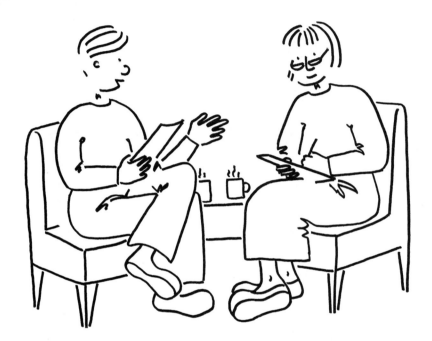

INTRODUCTION

The nature of the work with children and adolescents and their families is demanding, challenging and rewarding at times, but does evoke feelings of stress, distress and pain. The nature of the political climate of the wider working cultures of most organisations within the UK – be it health, social services, education or the voluntary sector – can also be stressful and painful. There will always be pressure of waiting lists and requests to see more people. There will always be frustration with having to carry out, at times, seemingly unrelated and unnecessary administrative duties.

Occupational therapists working in child and adolescent mental health services (CAMHS) may be fortunate to be within an occupational therapy department, but it is more likely that they will be working single handed in a department, isolated from other occupational therapists. It is also possible that their line manager will not be an occupational therapist or, if so, will have different clinical expertise and no experience of child psychiatry.

When working in isolation it is essential to address the issue of who is responsible for supervising and supporting the occupational therapist in the following areas:

- professional development as an occupational therapist
- everyday clinical practice
- managerial practice.

This chapter endeavours to address the importance and value of supervision and support by providing an overview of the aspects of supervision, in particular clinical supervision, and supportive systems. It aims to provide and remind occupational therapists of tools to assist in being proactive in looking after themselves and keeping themselves – and consequently others – safe.

DEFINITION OF SUPERVISION

The College of Occupational Therapy's statement on supervision highlights that supervision should be an interactive process through which the supervisee is assisted in professional and personal development and a means of ensuring that the supervisee is able to do their job effectively (College of Occupational Therapy 1997). Butterworth & Faugier (1992) describe it as 'an exchange between practising professionals to enable the development of professional skills'. Loganbill, Hardy & Delworth (1982) suggest it is an 'interpersonally focused, one to one relationship in which one person facilitates the development of therapeutic in the other person'. Inskipp & Proctor (1988) define it simply as 'extra-vision'.

The definition of supervision is very much determined by the tasks or functions that this interactive process is aiming to achieve. Defining clinical supervision brings other synonyms to mind such as mentorship, appraisal and teaching. These processes provide different qualities in assisting the development of the practitioner. In mentorship, an experienced practitioner models how practice could be, encourages the achievement of high standards, and promotes evaluation and reflection of clinical skills.

Appraisal (or individual performance review) is a two-way process involving the supervisor (who is usually the line manager) and the supervisee. In this, both parties systematically reflect on the performance of the supervisee; acknowledge achievements in their performance; and identify training and other development needs. It provides an opportunity to consider long-term career development. It should also enable the appraisee to have a better understanding of the manager, their expectations and those of the organisation. Clinical supervision can help to inform appraisals and can help to address the issues arising from appraisal.

In teaching, an experienced practitioner enables a supervisee/student to acquire skills through the encouragement of use of reflective practice, by demonstrating a skill and/or by formal instruction. Clinical supervision in CAMHS will often assimilate the approaches used in counselling supervision.

FUNCTIONS OF CLINICAL SUPERVISION

Being aware of the different functions of the term 'supervision' will assist you and your line manager in clarifying personal needs and in considering how to best meet these needs. Kadushin (1976) describes three main functions or roles:

1. Educative
2. Supportive
3. Managerial.

Proctor (1986) uses the same three categories but employs the terms:

- formative
- restorative
- normative

The educative or formative function   focuses on developing the skills, levels of understanding and abilities of the supervisee.

The supportive or restorative function   allows the supervisee to be aware of how the client's distress and pain is affecting them and how they can deal with their own and their client's reactions.

The managerial or normative function   focuses on developing a high quality of professionalism in working with people.

Holloway & Acker (1988) list five functions of supervision:

1. Monitoring and evaluating
2. Instructing and advising
3. Modelling
4. Consulting
5. Support and sharing.

THE BENEFITS OF SUPERVISION

The cost of supervision in terms of person-hours, energy and commitment can seem immense. Ownership by the supervisee and management will assist in ensuring supervision is varied and actually happens.

The people to gain from the practice of effective supervision are the client essentially, the supervisee, supervisor, the department and the wider organisation itself.

The client

The main reason for supervision is to benefit the client. Supervision should enable effective intervention by the professional and safeguard good quality. The intervention should ultimately lead to the empowerment of the client.

The supervisee

Supervision can enhance staff performance, alleviate stress and prevent 'burn-out'. Burn-out is a state of emotional and physical exhaustion, which affects the worker's attitudes and beliefs about themselves and their clients. Low morale, sense of failure, lack of concern for the job and the depersonalisation of clients can occur. Pines, Aronson & Kafrey (1981) describe burn-out being 'the result of constant repeated emotional pressure associated with an intense involvement with people over long periods of time'.

Therapists work more productively when they feel valued and acknowledged.

The supervisor

Supervision enables the supervisor to keep in touch with clinical practice and enables the continuation of the learning process through the reflective practice and the creativity that the supervisee brings to the session.

The service/organisation

Supervision increases staff commitment as it reflects the commitment by the organisation to their staff by acknowledging and affirming their value. It can influence the rate of staff turnover, sick leave and those leaving the profession altogether (Allan 1997).

Allan (1997) in her recent research concluded that, although not all the elements of supervision are significant in lowering individual stress levels, supervision tailored to the individual's need does have a major part to play in influencing stress levels. Less supervision correlated with higher stress and high stress correlated with the likelihood of staff leaving the profession. Butterworth (1997) infers that supervision improves the relationship between professional and client, between professionals, and between professional and manager.

Supervision enhances the organisation and promotes the use of personal and professional resources (Hawkins & Shohet 1989). It can offer an effective mechanism to help purchasers and providers of health care discuss and share practice (Butterworth 1997).

Cost implications are often at the forefront of most managers' thoughts. Effective supervision can also lead to reducing the length of intervention by:

- clarifying objectives
- continual evaluation of clinical practice by helping the therapeutic process to move on when it has become 'stuck'
- helping therapists end an intervention with a client – a common difficulty for many therapists, particularly when working with clients who have seemingly infinite needs.

THE SUPERVISORY RELATIONSHIP IN CLINICAL SUPERVISION

The importance of the supervisory relationship is emphasised by Hunt (1986): 'It seems whatever approach or method is used, in the end it is the quality of the relationship between supervisor and supervisee that determines whether supervision is effective or not'.

The supervisory relationship is more successful when the following have been considered:

- level of experience of the supervisee
- theoretical approaches of both
- supervisor and supervisee including views, values, beliefs, attitudes and assumptions to behaviour and change
- cultural characteristics including gender, ethnicity, race, sexual orientation, religious beliefs and values.

The supervisor's tasks

'Setting the scene' is essential. This important task of the supervisor in creating this is described succinctly by Proctor (1986): 'The task of the supervisor is to help him (the supervisee) feel received, valued, understood on the assumption that only then will he feel safe enough and open enough to review and challenge himself, as well as to value himself and his own abilities. Without this safe atmosphere, too, he is unlikely to be open to critical feedback or to pay good attention to managerial instruction'.

Holloway (1995, p. 2) describes the clinical supervisor as 'the translator of theory and research in practice' and that their task is to 'articulate the layers of thinking, understanding, conceptualising and applying'. The supervisor needs to acquire, as Hawkins & Shohet (1989) describe, a 'helicopter ability'. The supervisor needs to be able to switch perspectives, hovering between being focused on:

- the client
- the supervisee and the therapy process
- the supervisory relationship and how this reflects the therapy process
- enabling a view of the client as part of a larger system
- viewing the work in the wider context of organisation and inter-organisational issues.

As in therapy, the emphasis of the supervision should be on empowering the supervisee through the development of their practice.

The supervisee's tasks

Although an interactive and reciprocal process, much of the onus in ensuring supervision actually happens and in the way that is most helpful to the supervisee lies with the supervisee themselves. Planning and preparation enables the time to be used most effectively. In doing so the following tasks must be considered:

- Ensuring the environment in which supervision takes place is suitable, in particular that it is quiet, private and unlikely to be interrupted by people or phone calls.
- Protecting supervision time. 'If you value it, use it.' If the session needs to be cancelled, rearrange another time as soon as possible. It will be helpful to block book several sessions at a time. As in therapy, having a regular time for supervision does reinforce commitment and continuity.

- Preparing and identifying the particular practice issues you need to address.
- Monitoring and evaluating supervision with the supervisor. Acknowledging and sharing freely what works well and what is difficult.
- Being open to feedback.
- Reflecting on how the supervisee themselves reacts to feedback.
- Monitoring tendencies to justify, explain or defend and, if so, consider the reasons for this.
- Being aware of professional codes of conduct and practice.
- Being assertive, valuing oneself in ensuring personal professional needs are met.

CLINICAL SUPERVISION ARRANGEMENTS

There are many supervision arrangements. None is perfect at meeting all needs or surmounting potential anxieties or threats, but some may be more suited to specific work settings. Carroll (1996) has outlined the strengths and weaknesses of a range of methods, some of which are included here.

Self-supervision

This is a reflective form of monitoring practice and evaluating work systematically. It will be described in more detail later in this chapter. Most supervisors see this as preparation for supervision rather than a type of supervision. This should be a continual process. Although there are advantages, as it is inexpensive and timing can be flexible, there is a risk of losing objectivity and overlooking transference and countertransference issues.

Individual supervision (with supervisor from own discipline)

In this arrangement there is an identified supervisor who is an experienced practitioner. This offers a more personal approach, enabling particular skills used by the supervisor to be developed. However, it may seem threatening as the supervisee is the sole focus. A dependency on

the supervisor, who is seen as
created.

Individual supervision (with supervisor different discipline)

This arrangement is more likely to occur in CAMHS. There needs to be a common understanding of the theoretical approaches used and an acceptance of difference in professional perspectives.

Individual peer supervision (the supervisory role is taken in turns)

This form may be useful to consider if there is another CAMHS occupational therapist working locally. It is more suitable for more experienced therapists, and may be helpful in consolidating experience, theory and role identity, but competition needs to be controlled.

Group supervision within own discipline with one supervisor

This will be possible if working within a paediatric occupational therapy department. It will also be useful to use with paediatric occupational therapists from other areas (e.g. neurology, learning disability, orthopaedics), to maintain a holistic approach.

Group supervision in which supervisors are from different disciplines with one supervisor

A range of life, cultural, gender and clinical experiences is available for discussion. Trust may take time to develop and powerful group dynamics may prevent the work of supervision.

Peer group supervision

Members of the group are experienced in practice and fulfil the roles of supervisor and supervisee. Consideration needs to be made about how membership is agreed.

Team supervision

This focuses on the interpersonal and group issues that arise from working together as a team.

he supervisor is not a member of the team. Strengthening of the team's identity and commitment may be achieved by this method.

REFLECTIVE PRACTICE

Reflection achieves a better understanding of practice and enables practitioners to learn from their experience.

Reflection involves considering in detail the process of an interaction, the effects on emotions and behaviours of both the client and the therapist, the strategies used and alternative strategies that could have been used and what has been learnt from this experience.

Christopher John's Model of Structure Reflection (1994) provides a helpful format for self-questioning.

Description

- Write a description of the experience.
- Identify the key points within the experience that need attention.

Reflection

- What was I trying to achieve?
- Why did I intervene as I did?
- What were the consequences of my actions?
  – for the patient and family
  – for myself
- How did I feel about this experience?
- How did the patient feel about it?
- How do I know how the patient felt about it?

Influencing factors

- What internal factors influenced my decision-making and actions?
- What external factors influenced my decision-making and actions?
- What sources of knowledge did or should have influenced me?

Alternative strategies

- Could I have dealt better with the situation?

- What other choices did I have?
- What would be the consequences of these?

Learning

- How can I make sense of this experience in the light of past experience and future practice?
- How do I now feel about this experience?
- Have I taken effective action to support others and myself as a result of this experience?
- How has this experience changed my ways of knowing and understanding in practice?

Reflection allows time to stop, take stock, make sense of what has happened, consider alternative strategies, learn from our experiences and move forward.

WHAT MIGHT HAPPEN IN SUPERVISION

Having clarified that supervision has different functions and that there is a need to make these explicit and overt when organising the sessions, the content of the session also need to be addressed. This includes the style of supervision used and other learning tools to be used.

Supervision styles

Hawkins & Shohet's (1989) process model defines two styles of supervision:

1. Supervision focusing on the therapeutic session. In this, there is a reflection of content of the therapy session, exploration of strategies and interventions used by the therapist, and exploation of the therapy process and relationship.

2. Supervision addressing 'how the system is reflected in the here-and-now experiences of the supervision process'. In this, the issues around the therapist's countertransference, the parallel between the supervisory and therapy relationship, and the supervisor's countertransference are explored.

Hunt (1986) outlines three styles of supervision.

1. Case-centred approach

2. Therapist-centred approach in which the focus is on the behaviour, feelings and processes of the therapist.
3. An interactive approach, focusing on both the interaction in the therapy relationship and the interaction in the supervisory relationship.

Presentation styles

The method of presentation of material in supervision also needs clarifying at the 'setting-up stage'.

A résumé of information concerning the client is helpful. The content of this is the same as would normally be included in a case presentation: age, gender, family structure, family and social history, medical history, presenting problems, reason for referral, outline of intervention plan; involvement of other agencies; initial impressions and observations of the client. This is important material to use in beginning to understand the behaviour of the child and how the family members may be feeling, and to address the feelings, behaviours and beliefs that this information may evoke within the therapist.

The supervisee and supervisor may agree to use only verbal feedback based on a summary from a session, or they may decide that it is more helpful to have a written account of the whole session. Role-play, audio and videotapes may also be useful tools to consider in promoting more reflection and objectivity.

A decision will also be needed with regard to keeping records of the supervision session. Each organisation within which the supervisee is working may have official guidelines regarding this. An examples of a format used in recording clinical supervision is shown in Figure 14.1.

TRANSFERENCE AND COUNTERTRANSFERENCE

In CAMHS, particularly when using a psychotherapeutic model, the issue of transference and countertransference must be respected. Houston (1990) refers to this as listening to 'the echo within us'.

Transference

The feelings and reactions that clients impart to therapists are likely to lead to paralleling, i.e. taking on and owning the difficult feelings the clients are waiting to be rid of and avoid. If not addressed within supervision, the process may paralyse the therapist's ability to work with the client.

Countertransference

How we think, feel, react with our client in response to their transference is countertransference, and working with it is a useful therapeutic tool. Within countertransference, the therapist needs to be aware that:

- the client may evoke feelings within her that remind her of a past relationship or experience.
- the client may impose a role on the therapist, such as a parent, which the therapist may assume and replay the client's experience within the session.
- the therapist may resist or avoid the transferred role; for example, in order to avoid the mother role, the therapist may adopt a more masculine, brusque manner.

Although holding the client's intense difficult feelings of anxiety, rage or sadness can seem overwhelming, Hawkins & Shohet (1989) remind us that clients have often lived with this pain for many years and their ability to tolerate the pain is probably greater than the therapist's.

TIME ISSUES IN SUPERVISION

Supervision, its provision and frequency will be influenced by the philosophy of each individual unit, by individual needs relating to stage of professional development, and by how much the supervisee values it. In practice, the frequency for formal clinical supervision can vary from daily, weekly, fortnightly to monthly. To allow sufficient time for presentation and discussion of material, an allowance of at least an hour should be considered. Longer sessions may be more useful if meetings are monthly or at greater intervals.

SOUTHAMPTON COMMUNITY HEALTH SERVICES TRUST

OCCUPATIONAL THERAPY SERVICES

RECORD OF SUPERVISION

NAME   SUPERVISOR

DATE   TIMES – From   To

DATE OF LAST SUPERVISION

ISSUES CARRIED OVER FROM LAST SESSION:

NEW ISSUES TO BE RAISED THIS SESSION:

SUMMARY OF MEETING (main points of discussion, decisions made):

Staff Member Initials   Supervisor Initials

Figure 14.1   Example of a contract for clinical supervision (with thanks to K Edwards, Clinical Supervision Project, Southampton Community Health Services Trust, Tatchbury Mount, Calmore, Southampton SO40 2RZ, UK) © Southampton Community Health Services Trust 1997.

Monthly sessions may also be useful to consider rather than more frequent meetings, if travel time has to be taken into account.

Butterworth's (1997) evaluation of supervision found that an average individual supervision took 45 minutes and occurred at least monthly, and that group supervision took more time (1.5–2 hours), and also occurred at least monthly.

CONTRACTS

Contracts give clarity, credence and ownership, and need to be drawn up together (with both the supervisor and supervisee) before supervision begins. Carroll (1996) suggests that four areas need to be addressed in the contract:

1. The practicalities
2. The working alliance
3. Presenting supervision
4. Evaluation.

Practicalities

- Include frequency, duration of each session, venue.
- Allocation of time for each participant in group supervision will be agreed.
- Cost implications, for instance if the supervisor is bought in from another Trust or organisation, will also be clarified. Not paying may be a false economy.

The working alliance

- Roles and responsibilities of the participants
- How and when the alliance will be reviewed.

Presenting supervision

- How will supervision time be used?
- How will clients be presented (e.g. verbally or written or video, etc.)?
- Will notes from supervision be kept?
- Where will notes be stored?
- Should a record be made in patients' notes that supervision has occurred and include a summary of the supervision session?

Compiling a contract may initially appear to be pedantic, but it does save time in the long run and can iron out many difficulties and resolve different expectations before they hinder the process. An example of a contract is given in Figure 14.2.

ACCESSING SUPERVISION

Gaining support from the line manager. Having defined the need – whether it be clinical supervision regarding professional and educational development, or clinical supervision focusing on the psychodynamic process of clinical interventions, managerially focused support – the support of the line manager must be sought in the first instance. Refer back to the section on Benefits of supervision should a convincing tactic regarding its value be required.

Accessing clinical supervision to focus on the psychodynamic process. It is unlikely, due to lack of numbers, that the clinical supervisor will be an occupational therapist. Team members and colleagues may be able to recommend local supervisors.

Consider funding. It may be possible that the organisation will 'buy in' a clinical supervisor from another Trust or organisation. 'Buying in' an occupational therapist adviser when the line manager is not an occupational therapist is important to consider in order for professional identity and development to be maintained.

LINE MANAGEMENT SUPERVISION

This chapter has focused primarily on clinical supervision, but line management supervision must not be overlooked. As management skills are generic to all areas of occupational therapy, only general issues will be raised.

The aims of line management supervision are different and can include the following:

- to develop skills in workload management, priority setting, time management, teaching and working as a team member
- to explore and solve problems/issues causing difficulty

- to monitor professional standards of practice
- to identify personal development needs and facilitate personal growth
- to set personal goals and service objectives
- to identify the range of resources available to enable effective case work and personal growth through case supervision
- to discuss development and progress of the service.

The supervisee does not have a choice in selecting the line manager/supervisor and the relationship will be modified or terminated in relation to the work contract as opposed to having a time-limited relationship as in clinical supervision.

It is possible that the line manager will be from a different profession. The art of politics and how to influence people becomes more predominant in these interactions. The notion that managers do not understand or listen to the supervisee's needs is familiar, not just to occupational therapy. Integrating and creating a common language between the supervisor and supervisee can at times seem impossible.

Kakabadse (undated) refers to the need to identify the 'comfort zones' of those one wishes to influence. Comfort zones consist of behaviour, values, attitudes and ideas that an individual is able to accept, tolerate and manage. Together they form a person's 'identity' and will enable the supervisee to present their issues in a manner that is less threatening and which highlights the positive effects for the supervisor (i.e. identifying 'what's in it for them').

Line management responsibilities for the supervisee should be made explicit. The need for this is highlighted in the event of legal proceedings such as in complaints procedures or if the supervisee is expected to write court reports or give evidence in court.

It is useful to make a record of line management supervision sessions (see Fig. 14.2). Using a pro forma will assist in:

- using the session effectively
- empowering the supervisee in ensuring their particular issues are addressed as well as those of the supervisor

- recording any action agreed
- recalling discussions and agreed plans from previous sessions.

TIME MANAGEMENT

Managing time brings to mind taming a wild horse. Some of the time the rider feels in charge and in control of the horse's pace and direction but always alert and aware that the horse could suddenly buck and gallop off at any moment. Some of the time the rider might feel that the saddle has slipped and they are being dragged along underneath the horse and trying desperately to hold on. Most of the time we are just holding on, with some control at least of the direction in which we should be heading.

The following strategies may help to maintain control:

1. Boundary setting between work and leisure. The responsibility for boundary setting is yours. Do be flexible in your work hours if possible. There will always be clients who request later appointments. Remember, though, to ensure that there is a balance between work and home life.

2. Avoid squeezing in appointments over lunchtime. You do need this space. You cannot indefinitely continue to work through whole days without affecting standards of practice and causing yourself stress.

3. Booking appointments. Once you have planned your intervention, book all the planned number of sessions in your diary immediately including the review date with your colleagues. Coordinating diaries with colleagues can be a nightmare. It is easier to cancel appointments than to arrange them. Your diary will soon become full.

4. Booking administration time. Firmly block this out in your diary to make it difficult to write appointments in this slot. This will at least remind you that you need it (before reaching for the Tippex to squeeze in another appointment). Half an hour at the end of the day can achieve 'desk control' and 'head control', i.e. sorting out mail, small administrative tasks, phone calls, and

SOUTHAMPTON COMMUNITY HEALTH SERVICES (NHS) TRUST

CONTRACT FOR CLINICAL SUPERVISION

Name of supervisee   _____

Designation   _____

Discipline & Grade   _____

Base & Tel. No.   _____

Date of appointment   _____

Name of supervisor   _____

Designation   _____

Base & Tel. No.   _____

Model of supervision   _____

Period of supervision   _____

Length of session   _____

Frequency of sessions   _____

Venue for supervision   _____

Contract agreed between:

_____ (Supervisee)

_____ (Supervisor)

_____ (Supervisee's manager)

on   _____ (Date)

Figure 14.2   Example of a summary record of clinical supervision (with thanks to G Roder, Director of Occupational Therapy, Department of Rehabilitation, Southampton General Hospital).

The SUPERVISEE will be responsible for:

1 completing the supervision contract in consultation with the supervisor and the manager.

2 identifying personal supervision objectives which relate to professional development.

3 recognising relevant issues and information to bring to supervision.

4 being prepared to discuss these issues openly and honestly.

5 identifying and communicating to the supervisor the most useful type of response.

6 being open to feedback, including constructive criticism.

7 reflecting upon and learning from the process of supervision.

8 undertaking appropriate supportive activity outside the supervision session.

9 integrating the learning outcomes of supervision into professional practice.

10 keeping the manager informed of the progress with supervision.

The SUPERVISOR will be responsible for:

1 recognising their abilities and limitations in respect of clinical supervision.

2 assisting the supervisee to explore and reflect upon professional practice.

3 encouraging the supervisee to examine the attitudes, values, beliefs and experiences which underpin professional practice.

4 sharing information, knowledge, skills and experience relevant to the supervision objective with the supervisee.

5 giving open, honest and constructive feedback.

6 acknowledging and promoting good professional practice.

7   challenging aspects of practice in a sensitive and productive manner.

8   enabling the supervisee to recognise when there is a need to modify/develop existing practice or adopt new practices.

9   facilitating and supporting change.

10 identifying when an issue raised in supervision needs to be shared with a manager.

The SUPERVISEE and SUPERVISOR will be JOINTLY responsible for:

1   ensuring that the supervision arrangement is given priority status.

2   maintaining the confidentiality of the content of the supervision sessions, including any information relating to a third party.

3   keeping appropriate written records of the supervision.

4   reviewing the progress of the supervision at agreed intervals.

5   acknowledging and not transgressing the boundaries of supervision.

SOUTHAMPTON COMMUNITY HEALTH SERVICES (NHS) TRUST

Supervision objective (state date identified):

Supervision methods employed:

When will progress be reviewed?

What evidence will be used to demonstrate achievement?

enabling you to prepare (at least at an awareness level) for the next day.

5. Make lists of what needs to be done.
6. Prioritise items each day in the order:
   a) must be done today
   b) should be done today
   c) might be done today
7. Make phone calls in batches.
8. The greatest interrupter is you. Tackle one task at a time, finish it, then move on.
9. Handle paper only once.
10. Sort mail into:
   a) for attention and do straight away
   b) for information; read, file or throw away
   c) for waste.

CASELOAD MANAGEMENT

Weighting and prioritising

Jasinska (1991, 1992) gave practical advice in helping to manage present caseloads and prioritise new referrals. The system she created was to help define a therapist's personal maximum caseload, not to dictate a general time-table.

Calculating the number of clinical sessions

1. Review an average month and draw up four weekly timetables.
2. Divide the blank timetables into hourly slots.
3. Write in regular commitments:
   – meetings
   – general administration
   – study/research time
   – travel
   – caseload planning and write-ups
   – management duties
   – report writing

Jasinska also suggests including time spent for the previously unscheduled, but vital, parts of your job (e.g. time for developing assessment techniques).

4. Add up the number of free hours over a month.
5. Calculate the length of an average session, e.g.:

Session	50 minutes
Travel	15 minutes
Notes	15 minutes
Treatment planning and liaison	40 minutes
Total	2 hours

6. Divide the number of free hours by the length of an average session.
7. This will give you the maximum number of sessions an occupational therapist can do per month, for example:

No. of working hours per month = $36 \times 4 = 144$
No. of allotted hours = 44
'Free hours' = $144 - 44 = 100$
Divide the no. free hours by the length of an average session = $100/2 = 50$

Maximum no. of sessions per month = 50

Weighting your present caseload

This is a system to address your current caseload, but not your ideal caseload. It can also be used to calculate the deficit of hours in your service.

To help prioritise your clinical input, cases are 'weighted' according to the amount of input required, for example:

Weekly session	weighted 4
Fortnightly sessions	weighted 2
Monthly sessions	weighted 1
Bi-monthly sessions	weighted 0.5
Termly sessions	weighted 0.25

Jasinska points out that the system addresses an occupational therapist's current caseload but does not take into account the ideal weighting. She suggests addressing this by keeping a tally of the actual weighting a child receives and also that of the ideal weighting, for example:

Name	Age	Diagnosis	Actual weighting	Ideal weighting
J B	4	Depression	1 (monthly)	4 (weekly)

Weighting your waiting list

To help manage and prioritise new referrals and waiting lists, Jasinska (1992) suggests initially formulating a list of specific areas of concern that will ascertain level of urgency for each case that is sympathetic to the individual service. She gives the following examples:

- Optimum timing of intervention
  - What will be the effect of non-intervention or delayed intervention?
- Client, carer, parental anxiety
  - Is there an increased level of anxiety for the child, parent or carer, and would therapy ameliorate the situation?
- Effect on function
  - To what extent is the problem affecting the child's function?
- Client/carer's ability to cooperate with therapy
  - Is there a named person who will support the intervention and carry through any advice given?
- Expected outcomes
  - What difference will therapy make to the child and family?
- Availability of appropriately skilled staff
- Potential for change
- Other agencies involved
  - How much therapy input is the family already receiving?
- Age of child
  - Efficacy of intervention can depend on child's age, level of compliance, motivation, etc.
- Diagnosis – prioritising purely in terms of diagnosis does not recognise the varied needs each child has due to different individual circumstances.

Each concern is given a weight from 0 to 3, as follows:

3   most urgent – severe problem/effect
2   moderate problem/effect
1   mild problem/effect
0   not applicable/no effect

For example:

Optimum timing	3
Client, carer parental anxiety	0
Effect on function	1
Cooperation with therapy	1
Expected outcome	2

Availability of skilled staff	3
Potential for change	1
Other agencies involved	3
Age of child	1
Diagnosis	1
Total	16

The more points the case has, the more priority the case should receive. Jasinska (1991, p. 25) states that the system advocates the use of waiting lists: 'If paediatric occupational therapists continue to increase their caseload, without any monitoring system, the quality of their work is bound to deteriorate'.

SUPPORT AND NETWORKING

Supervision has a supportive role, but should not be deemed as the only support mechanism. Support in the workplace can be gained from a number of sources. Time-out arrangements, good communication, good management, peer support groups, in-service training courses, counselling services and occupational health have been outlined as broad elements of positive support systems by the National Association for Staff Support (1992).

Peer group support

Talking to colleagues, peer group support, life outside work and the family are other important factors in helping people cope with stress.

Lunchtimes and tea breaks are important times, not only to rest and refresh, but to meet and connect with colleagues. In-service training days not only meet the educational development but the social development of the team. Increasing understanding and awareness of how colleagues 'tick' is crucial in team building and support.

Environment

Environmental issues are acknowledged in interventions with clients. They should also be considered in enabling staff to function as a team. Lack of adequate office space and equipment creates unnecessary stress and time wasting that is realised only when these deficits are resolved.

The importance of having a main base should not be underestimated. It is important to be able to return to base, to fellow team members, who are important in providing a supportive environment. A base creates security. Accessibility of team members provides much more opportunity for cross-fertilisation of ideas, informal education sharing and for speeding up communication generally.

Professional organisations

In the UK, the National Association of Paediatric Occupational Therapists (NAPOT) provides an important starting point for networking with other occupational therapy colleagues. In 1997, networks of occupational therapists working in CAMHS were established within NAPOT. These networks are lively and supportive, and allow like-minded, enthusiastic occupational therapists, who are often working single handed, to share and address managerial, clinical and educational issues and explore joint initiatives in the areas of research and education.

Mapping your support system

Hawkins & Shohet (1989) provide a creative way to reflect on personal support systems.

- Take a large sheet of paper (A3 or bigger).
- In the middle, draw a picture or symbol of yourself.
- Around your symbol, draw pictures, symbols, diagrams or words to represent all the things and people that support you in being creative and in developing at work (e.g. walk to work, books you read, colleagues, meetings, friends, etc.).
- Consider the importance of these supports and your connection with them and try to represent this in your picture; for example, how strong are the links – tenuous and distant or very strong and regular? Do they support you from below as in strong foundations or are they balloons that lift you up? Are they near or far?

- With a different colour, draw symbols that represent those things that impede the use of these supports; for instance, fear of being criticised, unavailability, organisational issues.
- Share your picture with someone else – a supervisor, colleague, partner or friend.
- Ask them to respond to the overall picture: 'What impression does it create?'. Then discuss: Is this the kind of support you want? Is it enough? What sort of support is missing? How could you go about getting such support? What support is really positive for you to the extent that you must ensure that you nurture and maintain it? Which blocks could you do something about?
- Together try to develop some specific action plans from the discussion. These should include:
  - What are you going to do?
  - How are you going to do it?
  - When and where are you going to do it?
  - Who needs to help you?

CONCLUSION

Supervision and support are important in any field and at any level. When working in isolation, the occupational therapist needs to be even more proactive in accessing and attaining these.

In CAMHS, the main tools of therapy are the therapists themselves. Like tools, the therapist needs to be nurtured, valued, regularly maintained, overhauled occasionally, adapted to be in line with new models and respected to enable consistent safe and effective practice.

'There is a need to keep the intuitive self in repair' (source unknown).

REFERENCES

Allan F 1997 Once an OT, always on OT. College of Occupational Therapy, London

Butterworth T 1997 Clinical supervision: a hornet's nest? . . . or honey pot. Nursing Times 93(44):24–29

Butterworth T, Faugier J 1992 Clinical supervision and mentorship in nursing. Chapman & Hall, London

Carroll M 1996 Counselling supervision – theory, skills and practice. Cassell, London

College of Occupational Therapy 1997 Standards, policies and procedures. Statement on supervision in occupational therapy, SPP150(A). COT, London

Hawkins P, Shohet R 1989 Supervision in the helping professions. Open University Press, Buckingham

Holloway E 1995 Clinical supervision: a systems approach. Sage, California

Holloway E, Acker M 1988 Engagement and power in clinical supervision. Workshop presented at the Oregon Association of Counsellors Education and Supervision. Corvallis, Oregon

Houston G 1990 Supervision and counselling The Rochester Foundation, London

Hunt P 1986 Supervision. Marriage Guidance Spring:15–22

Inskipp F, Proctor B 1988 Skills for supervising and being supervised. Cited in: Hawkins & Shohet (1989)

Jasinska K 1991 Caseload management. NAPOT Newsletter Autumn:23–25

Jasinska K 1992 Prioritisation. NAPOT Newsletter Spring:18–20

Johns C 1994 Guided reflection – clinical supervision. A 1-day national conference, Birmingham

Kadushin A 1976 Supervision in social work. Columbia University Press, New York

Kakabadse A undated The politics of interpersonal influence. In: Managing health services, readings 10.1. Open Business School, Open University, pp 88–94

Loganbill C, Hardy E, Delworth U 1982 Supervision, a conceptual model. Counselling Psychologist USA 10(1):3–42

National Association for Staff Support 1992 Charter for staff support in the health care services. October

Pines A, Aronson E, Kafrey D 1981 Burnout: from tedium to growth. The Free Press, New York

Proctor B 1986 Supervision: a co-operative exercise in accountability. In: Marken M, Payne M (eds) Enabling and ensuring supervision in practice. Leicester National Youth Bureau, Leicester

FURTHER READING

Butterworth T, Carson J, White E 1997 It's good to talk. Manchester School of Nursing, Midwifery and Health Visiting, University of Manchester, Manchester

Hunter E 1997 Shifting the balance: empowering the occupational therapist through supervision. Paper presented to the College of Occupational Therapy conference, Southampton, UK, 1997 (c/o Edinburgh Health Care NHS Trust, Royal Edinburgh Hospital, Edinburgh EH10 5HF, UK)

Schon D 1983 Educating the reflective practitioner. Jossey-Bass, San Francisco

15

Protective legislation for children

Becky Durant

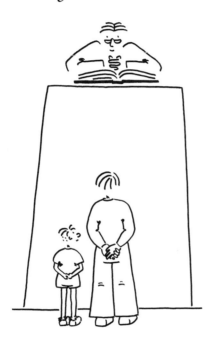

INTRODUCTION

Most people will have heard about the Jasmine Beck tragedy. Many will have experienced the flow of anger that swept through Britain following her death. Many wanted to point the finger at someone, others kept repeating: 'How did it happen? Why did it happen? It should never have happened.'

It is almost 20 years since the public outcry following Maria Colwell's death turned child abuse into 'legal property'. Previously the mistreatment of children behind closed doors was of little interest to lawyers or the legal profession as a whole. It became a concern for the courts only if a child died or was severely injured. Two further reports of child death inquiries, Kimberley Carlile and Tyra Henry, strengthened topical views that the law should be clarified and the powers of social workers increased. The inquiry following the Cleveland crisis turned attention to control of social work decision-making and, in particular, to the position of the courts. However, it was the proposals of the White Paper that accepted the recommendations of 'The Review of Child Care Law', set up by the then Department of Health and Social Security, on which the principles of the Children Act 1989 were finally based.

Now, every day of the week in courts, up and down the country, there are civil proceedings taking place designed to protect children from abuse. Specialist lawyers, judges and specialist police units are employed to identify and bring to trial cases where children have been abused by their adult caretakers.

The Children Act was born because current law appeared to be inadequate and failed to offer a clear and satisfactory framework for child protection.

This chapter describes and summarises aspects of the Act and law relating to children which might be helpful to occupational therapists (OTs) working with families. The purpose of the chapter is to raise issues and provoke thoughts, and also to indicate directions for further help and guidance. The author does not consider herself an expert in this very complicated field, but hopes the reader may find the chapter stimulating.

Two very important references worth mentioning at this stage are NHS Health Advisory Service (1996) and Dimond (1997). Bridget Dimond is a barrister who has also acted as a consultant and teacher at the College of Occupational Therapy. The book highlights the practical situations that may confront OTs and sets out succinctly the basic but relevant principles of law. It is a very useful reference book.

THE CHILDREN ACT

It was the intention of the Act to draw together public and private law and simplify existing legislation relating to children, in order to produce a more consistent code and strike a balance between family autonomy and the rights of children. Therefore, the Act introduced radical changes in the legislative base of childcare and has resulted in the most comprehensive changes in local authority care work for several decades. According to Lord Mackay (Hansard), it is 'The most comprehensive and far reaching reform of child law which has come before Parliament in living memory'.

The Children Act has considerable implications for childcare policies, practices and resources of social work and health service agencies. It makes a strong commitment to client participation and provides for a better framework of accountability than earlier legislation.

The Act is divided into 12 parts, each relating to a different aspect of child law. For purposes of this chapter, the focus will be on those parts that appear to be the most pertinent to OTs. However, the Act must be read as a whole, as the Lord Chancellor repeatedly stated during its passage through Parliament.

Main principles

1. The welfare of the child is the paramount consideration in court proceedings.
2. Wherever possible, children should be brought up and cared for within their own families.
3. Children should be safe and be protected by effective intervention if they are in danger, but this should be open to challenge by parents in the courts.
4. When dealing with children, courts should ensure that delay is avoided, and may make

an order only if to do so is better for the child than making no order at all.

5. Children should be kept informed about what happens to them and should participate when decisions are made about their future.

Parents with children in need should be helped by local authorities to bring up their children themselves. This help should be provided as a service to the child and his family and should:

- be provided in partnership with the parents
- meet each child's identified needs
- be open to effective independent representations and complaints procedures, and draw upon effective partnership between the local authority and other agencies, including voluntary agencies.

Local authorities are required to take a child's racial origin, culture and linguistic background, and religion into account when making decisions about them. So let's look at what these principles may mean and the implications they may have for practitioners.

Welfare is paramount

A child is anyone under the age of 18 years, but the court's power to make orders is restricted to those under 16, unless the case is exceptional. Case law will continue to suggest what the judiciary considers to be in the child's welfare. Psychological literature and other literature, including when appropriate OT recommendations, will provide a basis for argument.

The Lord Chancellor explained the new wording as follows:

the welfare of the child should come before and above any other consideration in deciding whether to make an order. (Herbert 1993, p. 208)

In the Act, the emphasis on the paramountcy of the child's welfare is as follows:

When a court determines any question with respect to the upbringing of a child or the administration of a child's property or the application of any income arising from it, the child's welfare shall be the court's paramount consideration.

Welfare checklist

The Act comes with a welfare checklist in order to facilitate consistency through the courts and across the country. It informs legal advisers and encourages those in dispute to concentrate on the issues that affect their children. It reads as follows:

a. the ascertainable wishes and feelings of the child concerned (considered in the light of the child's age and understanding)
b. the child's physical, emotional and educational changes
c. the likely effect on the child of any change in circumstances
d. the child's age, sex, background and any change in circumstances
e. any harm the child has suffered, or is at risk of suffering
f. how capable each of the child's parents, and any other person in relation to whom the court considers the question to be relevant, is of meeting the child's needs
g. the range of powers available to the court under this Act in the proceedings in question

IMPLICATIONS FOR OTS

The Act heavily emphasises the need for consultation, the importance of asking children for their views and their ideas. Some OTs may find themselves in the position of having to write a court report to help the advisers decide what may be the best interests of the child in relation to their upbringing. They may therefore need to work with the child in order to discover the child's views. This may represent a shift in therapy, a move a way from the original reason for referral, or it may come at the beginning of therapy and form part of an overall assessment package.

At the end of this chapter there is a discussion relating to interviews with children.

Communicating with the child is emphasised in the Act as the child's views are seen to be of great significance. Thus there is greater emphasis than in earlier legislation on consulting children and finding out their views. Instead of relying on the views of adults, the child will now be asked for his/her opinion but may well need the help of an OT to express it.

So, how do you find out what a child wants? Perhaps the main methods might include questions, listening and asking more questions, having first established a safe environment for the child to be able to communicate easily and confidently. We each have our own ways of creating this safe environment: some OTs use the familiar world of playrooms, others use art materials, whilst some may simply talk to the child without any toys. There really is no right or wrong way to do this; each therapist will have developed their own particular style of working. But one thing is certain: no therapist can possibly understand a child until they have formed a relationship, and this may take some time. This inevitably may lead to problems. Often, the courts want a decision to be made as quickly as possible as they do not consider that it is in the child's interest to be kept waiting.

So what does the therapist do when faced with a demand for an urgent court report? What does the therapist do when therapy has only just started and a relationship has not yet been made with the child? What does the therapist do when their secretary is on holiday or overworked and can't possibly type the report? And – a very big dilemma – is it in the child's interest for you as therapist to write a report?

The first response is to panic! What to do? If you agree to go ahead, just how do you do it? If this is your first court report – and with the consequential implication of a court appearance – the prospect may seem daunting. Hopefully, most therapists will be working in centres where they have access to other therapists who will be experienced in this area: social workers, doctors, maybe other OTs. So the first thing to do could be to find someone and talk to them, first about your own concerns and then about what to do. It all sounds pretty obvious, but so many people prefer to suffer silently, locked away in their own office lamenting the lost opportunity of that study day about writing reports – it didn't seem very relevant then!

There is always someone who can help, and the best thing to do is to ask. There may be someone who is an expert in the Children Act, so it is important to find out who is the best person to consult about this. Every unit has its own child protection procedures and it is vitally important that all OTs working with children are aware of these. There are usually annual study days relating to child protection issues and, again, it is vitally important that therapists are given the opportunity to attend these days and familiarise themselves with current law and local policies and practices.

It is a good idea to discuss the Children Act with colleagues and also to invite good outside speakers. In this way, the Act and procedures become familiar and workable. One very important thing is to ensure that there is access to legal advice when and where necessary.

Each child and family centre is different. However, many have consultant psychiatrists who specialise in child protection work and they often have good relationships with judges and the courts in general. The consultant may well be the best person to help; often, you can arrange an extension for the report, as the deadlines may be flexible.

Of course, there is another option. You may consider that it is not in the child's best interest to provide a report. Perhaps this will jeopardise therapy. If so, careful thought is needed about the decision. On the other hand, you may be the best person to give the child a voice. It is worth mentioning these issues and also the fact that, unless the OT receives a subpoena, the therapist is under no obligation to write a report.

Note-taking: useful reminders

The court may request a report on a child from anyone in the health services. This report will draw on the objective information contained in the child's notes. It is important to emphasise the word 'objective' because notes need to be very clear and very concise. These notes may at some time be used as a basis for a court report, so it is good practice to assume that all notes will at some stage be needed for purpose of report writing. This will establish a good habit, hopefully.

Every therapist has their own particular style of note-taking. Some write notes during therapy; others wait and write them up afterwards. There are pros and cons for both methods; when you do the notes is entirely personal, but everyone needs to remember the following:

- All notes must be written in black ink.
- All notes must be clearly signed by the author and include the author's professional status.
- All notes must include the exact date, including year and time.
- All notes must include a list of all the people present, including observers such as students.

CHILD PROTECTION

Child protection is an important area which needs to be mentioned, but the reader should consult further literature for more details as this chapter cannot cover such a wide topic in depth.

When an OT is concerned that a child may be being abused, physically, emotionally or sexually, they must act immediately. Each authority will have its own particular procedures but there will always be a named person – either social worker or psychiatrist – whom the OT must approach if there are worries. In other words, immediate action must be taken to ensure that any concerns are drawn to the attention of the appropriate person. Thus all OTs must be familiar with the procedure and provisions for child protection. It is not always clear when action is necessary, but the OT must put the safety of the child first.

In any unit there should be an agreed procedure for the management of child abuse cases. Also a forum should exist in each local authority to ensure cooperation between all the agencies involved in the protection of young people at risk; this is usually referred to as the child protection committee.

Each authority must maintain a child protection register which provides a record of all children in the area who are the subject of a child protection plan. It also ensures that the plans are reviewed every 6 months and provides a focal point of inquiry for staff who have concerns over a child and want to know whether they are the subject of a protection plan.

CHILD DEVELOPMENT

Without an understanding of this concept, the therapist will not be able to assess the 'normality' of a child or adolescent's behaviour. Please refer to Chapters 4 and 12 for further information. However, the following may be useful points to consider.

Life itself encapsulates development and changes and transitions. These dynamic features apply not only to individuals but also to families. Families change according to the stages of development of all their members – children and adults. Some changes are expected, others are not. Some mercurial changes in behaviour are responses to the rapid growth, and the successive changes in life are difficult to identify at the onset. Each of us is unique, although it has been said that we are like all other persons, like some other persons, and like no other person. (Herbert 1993, p. 54).

ADOLESCENCE

The Act emphasises choice and the right to consent. Thus, it is important to understand how complicated life is for young people between the ages of 12 and 18 years. It is probably true to say that in the past half century or so adolescence in Western society has grown and lasts longer than before. This must reflect the confusion we have about deciding when a young person is sufficiently mature to make decisions and take responsibility. Society seems to be in a muddle because of the different ages required to leave school, smoke, drink and buy alcohol, manage a bank account, get married, drive a car, drive a motor bike, vote or be held responsible for a criminal act. At the time of writing, this the last point is under review, and children as young as 10 years may be considered responsible. So will adolescence be shortened? Or will the process of childhood lead swiftly into adulthood with no daylight in between?

But, if the Act encourages adolescents to make choices, the child's choice may depend on what is available. In the famous English case of Gillick v West Norfolk Health Authority (1985), for example, the children's right to contraception and contraceptive advice won through the courts would be meaningless if there were no services available to offer this advice. Similarly a child cannot decide to stay in a foster home if there are no long-term foster homes available.

It is worth mentioning the three points made by the Gillick judgement (Black et al 1989).

1. Parental powers are for the protection of the child.
2. Parental powers dwindle as the child matures. Lord Scarman said:

Parental rights yield to the child's right to make his own decisions when he reaches sufficient understanding and intelligence to be capable of making up his own mind on the matter requiring decision. (Black et al 1989, p. 76)

3. Parental powers depend on the understanding of the individual child, not on any fixed age.

Thus, young people under 16 years of age may be able to consent to treatment or indeed refuse it, depending on the situation. The person treating them has a responsibility to form a judgement upon their capacity to do this.

An example relating to the above frequently happens when a general practitioner refers a young person to an outpatient child and family department in confidence: in other words, without the knowledge or consent of the parent. In practice, this can prove difficult and cumbersome especially if the department has to send letters to a third intervening person, possibly the school. It may be helpful in this instance to look at the need for confidentiality and what it really means for the young person to keep their appointments secret.

OTHER ISSUES RELATING TO CONFIDENTIALITY

Consent to disclosure of confidentiality is essential, and without such consent disclosure would be unlawful. The patient should be competent to give consent and so, once again, it is difficult to define competency when dealing with young people. Where the child is aged under 16 years, the princi-

ples of the Gillick case would apply (see Dimond 1997, Ch. 23). However, it is essential to provide evidence that permission has been given, and some units may have their own forms for people to sign and date, authorising this permission.

Dimond illustrates a case of a mother who refuses care for herself when she probably needs it to look after her child successfully. She forbids the OT to discuss her needs with colleagues. In this instance it could be emphasised to the mother that action may have to be taken under the Children Act to secure the well-being of the child.

CHILDREN'S RIGHTS AND THE LAW

A big problem for the promoters of children's rights and autonomy is that what the child wants may not be what the law wants. Children may be removed from their homes in cases of child abuse because the situation does not seem safe for the child, but the child may not have been consulted or indeed have agreed to the idea. These are very difficult issues and, when these matters are discussed with the children, it is always hard to know how much influence they really have on the course of events – or indeed should have. How much should be determined by the professionals involved?

Box 15.1 illustrates the complexities of giving a child a voice.

Box 15.1

Following an initial assessment session with a child in foster care and also a session with the child's natural father, the OT wrote to the social worker outlining the content of the session and describing the explicit wishes of the father and son. In this instance both parties were very clear that neither wished to live with the other and both wanted the boy to stay with foster parents. The social worker replied swiftly clearly stating her position and views, which were contrary to the wishes of the family. She wanted the therapist to work with the father and son, to improve their relationship and maybe spend some weekends together.

In such an instance, how can workers juggle and compromise everyone's wish whilst remembering that the 'welfare and wishes of the child are paramount'?

Although some children may be mature enough to make decisions and choices, it takes much courage and perseverance on the child's part to resist the pressures from the legal machine. The right to choose imposes considerable responsibility on the child and adolescent. How can a child decide with whom they want to live, especially when they have equal fond memories of both parents? This often causes severe conflicts of loyalty as well as feelings of guilt towards the unchosen parent. If children are to be given rights, perhaps it should be the right *not* to choose and to have the responsibility of parents thrust upon them. Surely most children want to hear from their parents that they want the child? To put the child in the position of separating or divorcing a parent seems somewhat unfair.

THE MENTAL HEALTH ACT 1983

In certain circumstances this Act may be used to admit a young person to hospital as there is no age restriction on detentions under the Mental Health Act. Any person, on the application of an approved social worker or nearest relative and supported by two medical recommendations, may be detained in hospital under section 2 of the Act for up to 28 days. It must be considered that the person is:

- suffering from a mental disorder of such a degree that warrants detention of the patient in hospital for assessment and maybe medical treatment; or
- the person needs to be detained in the interests of their own health or safety or with the view of protecting others.

According to Dimond (1997), although the emphasis of the Act seems to be on compulsory admission and treatment, the reality is that this is avoided if alternative treatment and care is available outside. Often in cases of anorexia nervosa it is hoped to avoid using the Act and to persuade the young person and their family to agree to a voluntary admission. This is a difficult area and may cause problems in child and family units.

In Child and Adolescent Services, Safeguards for Young Minds, there is an informative and useful section on choosing between the Children Act 1989 and the Mental Health Act 1983 (NHS Health Advisory Service 1996, p. 87). In Dimond's book there is a very brief description of the Act and its implications for OTs (Dimond 1997, Ch. 21).

RIGHTS AND NEEDS

The use of courts and law to protect children's rights may be difficult and lead to problems. Are the rights of children the same as their needs? As mentioned above, the courts may be unable to protect children's rights because they do not have control over the resources on which those rights depend. At times it seems as if the use of law and powers of the legal system to force others to take account of the rights of the child may cause more problems than perhaps leaving matters as they are.

Parents who divorced 3 years ago may still be fighting over residency and access issues. Children are in the middle of a legal battle and may have to visit parents as determined by the existing court order and not when it feels naturally right or even convenient.

So, the operation of the legal process in children's cases may create more problems than it solves. Occasionally people become very entrenched in their positions. They reject the idea of compromise because it represents a loss of face. Sometimes it would be much easier if couples could reach their own agreements without the need for recourse to the law.

By structuring as a legal contest the emotional tangle that often follows the break up of close relationships, the law may succeed in channelling and so managing the conflict. In doing so, however, it allows the hostility and acrimony to find expression and feed upon the many opportunities that the legal process itself offers for humiliating, outwitting and defeating the once-loved-and-now-despised former partner or the once-helpful-and-now-interfering social worker. (King & Trowell 1992, p. 112)

Sometimes advice may be rejected by magistrates, who may not be as highly trained or qualified as the group of professionals employed to offer the advice. Another thought concerns crucial decisions about the future of children depending to a certain degree on the quality of the lawyers who appear in court or on the knowledge of part-time lay magistrates. Is it perhaps sometimes better for problems to be dealt with in a way other than bringing in the law and courts?

COURTS

There are a number of different courts that deal with factors relating to children:

The Youth Court. This deals with young offenders.

The Magistrates' Court. Under the Children Act a family panel of magistrates has powers to deal with family issues in the family proceedings court. They have jurisdiction to make orders concerning children and those relating to adoption, maintenance and domestic violence between spouses.

The County Court. Care proceedings from the magistrates' court are sometimes allocated to the County Court because of their complexity.

The High Court. Family matters are dealt with in the Family Division either at the Royal Courts of Justice in London, or at a district registry. They hear complex cases under the Children Act and also cases relating to adoption wardship and appeals from the magistrates' court.

The Court of Appeal. Appeals from the High Court and county court go to the Court of Appeal.

The House of Lords. This is the final court of appeal in the UK and will hear cases only when there is an issue of public importance.

(For further explanation of courts, see NHS Health Advisory Service 1996.)

THE LAW

The law can at times be very useful to set limits for acceptable parental behaviour and, of course, this in turn protects and looks after children.

Procedural rights

These are rights that look after children in the decision-making process but do not actually affect decisions. For instance, they include the right to have a voice and to express an opinion on

any matter that concerns the child's future welfare. In some formal decision-making processes they may require an adult to represent the child. OTs are often required to attend case conferences, and may well be the best person to represent the child's views.

Expert witness

OTs are often called upon to give evidence in court for a variety of different reasons. This section briefly highlights some of these areas.

There is an increase in the number of cases in which patients are seeking compensation for harm that may have occurred following injury, abuse, or a wide range of different situations. Inevitably this has led to the likelihood of the OT giving evidence in court.

OTs have particular skills in assessment, which means that their evidence is relevant in a wide range of court and tribunal hearings. Dimond (1997, Ch. 13) explores this in great detail. She discusses statement making, witness of fact, report writing and expert witness. In particular she makes some very sound and helpful suggestions about giving evidence.

Dimond (1997, p. 145) defines an expert witness as: 'someone who is invited to give evidence on any issue which is subject to dispute'. This may include an opinion about the outcome and prognosis of a patient where there is an argument over compensation.

According to Dimond, OTs have to honour their views and not vary or modify them according to the side that calls them. In any case, if an OT gives an honest view it must be easier to withstand cross-examination because they will be confident in their ideas and have evidence to support their views.

Useful suggestions for the expert witness are given by Dimond (1997, p. 147).

THE EDUCATION ACT 1993

As many children now have to go through the statementing procedure before they receive special help, it may be worth mentioning this Act briefly with reference to the report that an OT may need to provide. This Act came into effect in 1994 and placed duties on local education authorities to provide suitable education for children who are unable to attend school. A child has special educational needs if he or she has a learning difficulty. This basically means they have greater difficulty learning than the majority of children their age. It could also mean that they have a disability or illness that prevents them from attending school.

The Act contains duties to identify, assess and provide for those with such needs, which may involve a multidisciplinary assessment in collaboration with parents.

Children suffering from chronic conditions may benefit from a home tutor, but it may not be necessary to go through the statement procedure. The OT may need to write to either the coordinator of the visiting teacher department or the education department (depending on the policy of each area) to request home tutoring. Normally a very brief letter is sufficient, stating that the child is attending for treatment and not able to attend school for the moment. Permission to write must, of course, be sought from parents or carers.

Where an education authority considers that a child has special educational needs, the authority must carry out an assessment under section 167 of the Education Act. The authority will then be able to determine the special education provision necessary for the child. They have to inform the parents and explain the procedure, and also invite the parents to submit written evidence to the authority.

Under schedule 9 of the Act, the authority is required to seek medical, psychological and educational advice in connection with the assessment. Normally all professionals who have been involved with the child will be invited to submit a report. It should be remembered that the reports can be read by anyone who has been invited to submit one.

Finally, as many therapists working with children may find themselves in the role of the investigative interviewer, it is worth looking at some of the relevant issues that may arise in this context.

GENERAL POINTS TO REM WHEN 'INTERVIEWING' C

First, the OT needs to consider the differe between an investigative interview and a therapeutic interview, or indeed, in some instances, consider the similarities.

The word 'interview' is used with caution. Therapist may suddenly find themselves in the investigative interview situation, as well as a therapeutic session with a child. It may not be possible to separate the two, especially if the child thinks they are coming for therapy. Children are unable suddenly to switch into 'being interviewed' mode. Indeed, if the therapist suddenly changes the approach normally used in sessions, the child may become very confused.

Young children tend to be very talkative and the therapist needs to find a way to give the child an opportunity to talk about experiences. Adolescents may be more introspective – and are very good at using monosyllables when asked direct questions.

Children have a natural way of communicating through their behaviour and also through fantasy. Therefore, it makes sense for the therapist to find out how the child behaves and also to enter their fantasy world. Children interview in a different way from adults. They fidget, they change the subject, they are easily distracted, their concentration span is short, and they are much slower in their thoughts and verbal expression than grown-ups.

Children are not very good at answering questions related to their own feelings but they are good at describing things, and in particular relating how other people reacted and how they think other people felt. It is harder for them to say how they feel.

If therapists are going to use questions, these need to be short and easy to understand. The double-barrelled question, when two different answers are required, baffles all children and adolescents too. Also, it is important to remember when a child does not reply that they may not know the answer: they are not necessarily just being defensive or guarded.

Sometimes it is difficult for children to answer questions relating to their family because they may feel they are being disloyal. What is important is for the therapist to remember how the child responded. How did they react? What were the non-verbal messages? It may be necessary to include this in the report, to give a desciption of the child and their physical responses as well as verbal replies.

When a child is obviously having difficulty talking about possibly painful events in the family, it may be a good idea to make use of stories. The therapist could make up the main points of the story and leave gaps for the child to complete. From very simple beginnings, the therapist can gradually introduce different ideas such as fears, secrets, family arguments, behaviours, and so on.

PLAY AND BEHAVIOUR

Sometimes therapists use toys with children to help them describe what has happened to them. Animals, dolls, sand, anything with which a child may feel comfortable, can be used. Their play may indicate past sexual abuse. However, when children use toys to depict aggressive or sexual scenes, therapists have to remember that, on its own, this is not evidence of sexual abuse. Indeed, children often copy what they have seen on television or videos, or maybe they have witnessed sexual play in the home.

Children can be explicit in their play and may invite the therapist or interviewer to join in. Sometimes it can be very distressing and difficult to handle, especially if the child rubs themselves against the therapist or tries to touch the therapist's genitalia. It is always difficult to understand exactly what is happening. Is the child going through a phase of discovery? Are they engaged in explorative play with friends or even siblings? How much have they seen on videos? For the interviewer, it is very hard to unravel without making the interview abusive in itself. Many children engage in highly detailed sexual play but may not have been abused themselves.

Others are far less explicit in their play or may not play at all. It is important to record exactly and precisely what the child does and also to remember to ask the child to comment on their play too. Children like to talk but sometimes therapists inadvertently undermine their ability and focus exclu-

sively on non-verbal means of expression. It is fair to say that, by and large, children want to please adults. Therefore, they will respond in whatever way they think the adult wishes them to. If you put them in a room with paint and paper, they will probably paint. Likewise, if you put them in a room with constructional toys, they will play with the toys. If you take them to a sitting room with sofa or comfy chair, even the very young child will sit reasonably quietly and talk to you.

I think it is fundamentally important to help children to have a voice. The Children Act encourages collaboration with children. Today we are more aware of abuse. We need, as therapists, to be aware constantly of how we can enable children and adolescents to have a voice. We need to create the right climate in which the young person can express themselves freely and without fear of reprisal.

The search for the mechanisms to give children the opportunity to speak is easier than the practice of these mechanisms!

REFERENCES

Black D, Wolkind S, Harris Handriks J 1989 Child psychiatry and the law. Royal College of Psychiatrists, London
Dimond B 1997 Legal aspects of occupational therapy. Blackwell Science, London
Gillick v West Norfolk Health Authority 1985 2WLR, 830, House of Lords
Herbert M 1993 Working with children and the Children Act. British Psychological Society
King M, Trowell J 1992 Children's welfare and the law. The limits of legal intervention. Sage Publications, London
Lord Mackay. Hansard, H.L. vol. 502, col. 488
Lord Mackay. Hansard, H.L. vol.502, col. 1167
NHS Health Advisory Service 1996 Child and adolescent services, safeguards for young minds. HMSO, London

FURTHER READING

Brown S 1991 Magistrates at work. Open University Press, Buckingham

Levine M, Howard J 1995 The impact of mandated reporting on the therapeutic process. Sage Publications, London

Masson J 1990 The Children Act 1989, text and commentary. Sweet & Maxwell, London

Rosenbaum M, Newell P 1991 Taking children seriously – a proposal for a children's rights commissioner. Gilbenkian Foundation

Index